6 WEEKS TO A
HOLLYWOOD BODY

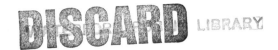

6 WEEKS TO A HOLLYWOOD BODY

Look Fit and Feel Fabulous with the Secrets of the Stars

STEVE ZIM AND MARK LASKA

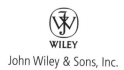

John Wiley & Sons, Inc.

Photographs by Nick Horn

Published by John Wiley & Sons, Inc., Hoboken, New Jersey
Published simultaneously in Canada

Design and composition by Navta Associates, Inc.

The information in this book is not intended to serve as a replacement for professional medical advice. Any use of the information in this book is at the reader's discretion. The author and the publisher specifically disclaim any and all liability arising directly or indirectly from the use or application of any information contained in this book. A health care professional should be consulted regarding your specific situation.

For general information about our other products and services, please contact our Customer Care Department within the United States at (800) 762-2974, outside the United States at (317) 572-3993 or fax (317) 572-4002.

Wiley also publishes its books in a variety of electronic formats. Some content that appears in print may not be available in electronic books. For more information about Wiley products, visit our web site at www.wiley.com.

Library of Congress Cataloging-in-Publication Data:

Zim, Steve.
  6 weeks to a Hollywood body : look fit and feel fabulous with the secrets of the stars / Steve Zim and Mark Laska.
       p.   cm.
    Includes index.
  ISBN-13 978-0-471-71549-8 (cloth : alk. paper)
  ISBN-10 0-471-71549-2 (cloth : alk. paper)
  1. Exercise. 2. Physical fitness. 3. Bodybuilding. 4. Nutrition. 5. Celebrities—Health and hygiene. I. Laska, Mark. II. Title.
    RA781.Z536   2006
    613.7—dc22   200519104

Printed in the United States of America

10 9 8 7 6 5 4 3 2 1

In memory of Cookie Zimelman

Contents

Acknowledgments

Thanks to my editor, Tom Miller, for shepherding this book; to Mark Laska, for making my words and ideas clear so that people can change their lives; and to Maria Yip for all the hard production work she puts into the fitness segments we do on NBC's *Weekend Today* show, which has helped spread the word of fitness to millions of people and has allowed me a forum to educate Americans on being healthier. To the gym crew—Salter Giddens, the gym's "fashion king"; Todd Bresler (or TT, as we call him); Chris Yackley; Diana Oliveira; and Kim Halcomb— thank you for always doing your best. Thanks also to Dennis Weiss for being a sounding board and keeping the gym healthier with all your fruit. Thanks to Chuck Dalaklis, Teresa McKeown, and the Brokaw brothers—your support has meant a lot to me. Thanks to Mel Berger and everyone at William Morris for finding us a good match. I also want to thank Dr. Abraham Zimelman—my dad and medical adviser for my fitness segments—and Dr. Alice Zimelman, Irv Rubinstein, and Shirley Rubinstein for being more than family and always coming up with ideas for me to do on the show. Thanks to my wife, Jodi, for everything she does—too much to list; to Carli and Taylor, my youngest workout buddies; and to Humphrey, my four-legged jogging partner. Thanks to Tom's editorial assistant, Juliet Grames; the book's production editor, Lisa Burstiner; and the copy editor, Mary Dorian. And finally, thanks to the models featured in the book who allowed us to show you the way: Ilana Zimelman, Marie Cavanaugh, Alyson Sanders, Amy Ruka, and Jodi Zimelman.

Introduction: What Is the Hollywood Body?

Within these pages you will learn the secrets of transforming your body into a Hollywood body. I have helped so many people through this process—people of all ages, shapes, and sizes—that it has been honed into a scientific formula that I am honored to share with you.

Around the world, Hollywood projects images of beautiful people, glamour, and star power. But the reality is somewhat different. People in southern California are blessed with one thing many other people are not: nice weather. People who visit Hollywood from Saskatchewan, Wisconsin, Maine, and North Dakota learn that they can actually enjoy being outdoors in February. In fact, most people in Hollywood are not that much better looking than people anywhere else in the world; we're just more active.

The Hollywood body is a product of an active lifestyle and a Hollywood body mindset. When you engage in activity, there is a natural release of hormones, enzymes, and chemicals that delivers instant feelings of well-being. Activity results in an immediate relief of stress; you will feel refreshed, energized, clearheaded, and buoyant—that is the Hollywood body mindset. These are the feelings that will drive you to become more active, and consequently, adopt an active lifestyle.

An active lifestyle will equate to a happy life. Happiness is actually the realization that you would not choose to be anyone or anything else. That is really the goal here. The point is not to look like your favorite celebrity, but to make the most of what you have. This book will help you change your body into the best that it can be— and be satisfied with who and what you are.

Let's be real: most of us do not look like supermodels or compete in bodybuilding contests. Recent studies conducted by scientific and medical institutions point out that less than 10 percent of the U.S. population exercises regularly. The Centers for Disease Control recently stated that more than 30 percent of the population is obese and more than 60 percent of all Americans are overweight. So Hollywood might not be the best litmus test for what your body could or should look like. During the press tour for the film *Bridget Jones: The Edge of Reason*, Renee Zellweger talked about "ballooning up" to 135 pounds. To put that in perspective, the average American woman weighs 162 pounds.

This book does not contain some unrealistic method to take a woman who is currently a size 26 and turn her into a size 2, or reduce a man's 42-inch waist to 28 inches. This book is designed for the great majority of people who do not exercise and would like to turn their lives around. If this is you, you are in the right place.

I have been an ardent fitness devotee my entire life and have been helping people transform their bodies for almost twenty years. I first began to take the transformation process seriously when I was in college. After watching people exercise next to me in the gym day after day and year after year, I began to notice that they looked no different from the way they did when I first met them. I began to question why and how these people could be so committed and not get any payoff for all their sweat and effort. I dissected the traditional exercises most of us are familiar with and became increasingly determined to discover the answer to why my gym mates were not getting results.

I began to study physiology; I delved into the function of supportive muscle groups, the skeletal system, kinesiology, and human performance. At a college in Boston, I was lucky enough to be allowed to observe some astounding scientific experimentation with next-generation magnetic resonance imaging (MRI) and infrared imaging that are considered cutting-edge technology. With advanced MRI technology, I could see how our muscles connect to the skeletal system and better understand their functions. On a hunch, I asked to see what muscles looked like during traditional exercises using infrared technology. It was clear that only a small portion of designated muscles were radiating enough heat to be seen. With this technology, it became evident that only 20 to 30 percent of the working muscle was actually being utilized.

Finally, I saw scientific proof that solved the mystery of why traditional exercises were not helping people transform their bodies. I began to modify traditional exercises and experiment with the creation of entirely new exercises to maximize muscular output, and I brought these new exercises back into the laboratory. The infrared images from the new exercises showed me that I could call upon 100 percent of muscular output. Theoretically, the new exercises provided a method to work the entire muscle and rebuild the musculature from its deepest point, giving exercisers a method to completely transform their appearance. When used in conjunction with proper nutritional guidelines and cardiovascular activity, the new exercises could result in a complete physical transformation in the shortest possible time.

After experimenting on myself and experiencing astounding results, I began working with high-level college athletes using these new techniques and methods. By anyone's definition, their results were off the charts. When I moved to Los Angeles, I began using these same techniques with professional and Olympic athletes. The system I developed has helped dozens of minor leaguers break into the majors, and it has propelled a handful of major league players to become all-stars. It has helped boxers to become world champions and amateur athletes to become national champions and Olympic medalists. It has enabled people to reach higher levels of performance after career-threatening injuries. In the sports world, the secret is definitely out, and several teams and organizations have instituted this system.

I own and operate a low-key private training center in Los Angeles. My clientele is an interesting mix of celebrities, professional athletes, and everyday folks who live in the neighborhood, including homemakers, merchants, civil servants, white-collar professionals, and entertainment executives, old and young. In this unpretentious environment, a sixty-year-old fire chief can stand next to a young ballplayer and say to himself, "If I work really hard, I can look like that." It is a place where a national champion figure skater will encourage a woman who has just had her second child to push herself on the next set of exercises. The majority of athletes I train are not seven feet tall and don't look like the Incredible Hulk; rather, they have well-toned and highly trained bodies. For the noncelebrities and nonathletes who come into my facility to make significant appearance- or health-related changes, the improvement happens rapidly and dramatically.

For the last few years, I have been talking publicly about the Hollywood body system. I have written over a hundred articles for magazines such as *Glamour*, *Cosmopolitan*, *Men's Fitness*, *Elle*, *Self*, *Redbook*, *Muscle & Fitness*, *Marie Claire*, *Oxygen*, and *ESPN*. I am the regular fitness expert on NBC's *Weekend Today* show, where I discuss fitness trends and health-related advances. On other networks, I have done dozens of nationally broadcast makeover features taking famous and not-so-famous people through the process of physical transformation on such shows as *Extra* and *Entertainment Tonight* and on VH1 and the Discovery Channel. The dramatic before-and-after stories of these celebrities have generated greater interest in this system, which I now have the privilege of bringing to you.

While these celebrities and athletes come into my gym to get a Hollywood body, I have designed this book so that you can get similar results in the privacy of your own home.

The Hollywood body workouts are designed to get you optimal results in the quickest possible time. Most people who stop exercising do so because they do not see results, but with the Hollywood body workouts your results are guaranteed. After just one workout you will feel the difference, after three workouts you will see the difference, and after only two weeks your friends and loved ones will notice the difference. After you have completed my six-week program, it is likely you will get a jaw-dropping reaction from everyone.

6 Weeks to a Hollywood Body is designed to take you from where you are to the results you have only dreamed about. I truly hope you will use this book, get the results you want, and feel comfortable enough to go to the beach and the gym, partake in fun and healthy activities, and take your fitness to the next level. By changing your body, I believe you will change your self-perception, your self-image, and your level of self-empowerment. Keep this in mind: changing your body will change your entire life!

Are you ready to get your own Hollywood body? Let's get started.

1

Hollywood Body Goals and Motivation

We spend significant portions of our free time watching television and movies. We gawk at the stunning female and male beauties on the screen. Film and television have defined our sense of beauty, and they powerfully project those standards and ideals. Whether or not we are conscious of it, celebrities are the very people with whom we compare and contrast our appearance. This book is devoted to the journey of how you get from where you are today to the body you would like to have in the future. That road can be littered with potholes and detours, and I will do my best to make sure you avoid these road hazards.

Unrealistic Expectations

A Hollywood body is not a *perfect* body. Trying to achieve a perfect body is the biggest and most common trap you can fall into; there is no such thing. Although a person's body can be beautifully sculpted and toned, no one has a perfect body. Even celebrities will blushingly point out their shortcomings—at least as they perceive them. The perfect body is impossible to achieve; it's simply unattainable.

Trying to achieve an unattainable goal is an exercise in futility. Although I would love to be 6'7", I will never be taller than 5'11". That is just the way it is. The point of this book is *not* about becoming someone else. There is no power in that. There is, however, power in becoming the best you can be. By merely *attempting* to make what you have the best it can be, you will become empowered.

Immediate Results

Improving your appearance, becoming fit, and being more physically active are the quickest and most surefire ways to increase your confidence, self-esteem, and self-worth. That is your ultimate payoff.

You need to make the payoff more immediate than a smaller dress size or the ability to run a marathon. This system of exercise must make you feel so incredibly good and so good about yourself that you would never even consider missing a workout. If you get a payoff each and every time you exercise, if you get many results every day, you will stick with it long enough to reach that final destination.

Positive Addiction

I want you to get something profound, something that will rock your world, every day. To do that, this program has a built-in mechanism to provide you with moment-to-moment results. As you will discover in the chapters that follow, the road map for a Hollywood body is a three-part system. I will give you a prescription for nutrition, cardiovascular exercise, and specific sculpting routines for your individual body type. At the beginning of each day, you will set yourself up to achieve many small personal victories. Every time you follow my nutritional guidelines, for example, you will have accomplished something tangible—it will become a personal victory. When you do your cardiovascular exercises, you will get many immediate results that include greater levels of energy, improved concentration, and feelings of well-being that may be more effective than antidepressants. These are personal victories as well. Throughout your sculpting routines you will be completely focused on each exercise repetition; each repetition that is performed to perfection is a personal victory. At the end of any given session, you will have achieved hundreds of minivictories.

These victories are the basis for your physical and personal transformation. Accumulating them daily gives you immediate results and the momentum to carry you through the day. This positive momentum propels you forward. No matter what is happening at home, in the office, or in your relationships, this positive momentum will affect almost every aspect of your life. It will compel you and drive you. In creating this incredibly positive force, you will have found the ultimate reason to use this system day after day. After only a week or two, instead of asking, "How can I find the time?" you will be saying, "How can I *not* find the time?"

Allowing Yourself Time

Forming a habit takes a specific amount of time. Behavioral scientists and 12-step programs have determined that it takes at least three weeks to break a negative habit and form a good one. This program is designed specifically to enable you to develop this habit.

To begin your personal journey of positive addiction, you need to set aside 45 minutes of your day three times a week. Before we go any further, get out your organizer, consult the nearest calendar, or log onto your computerized scheduling device. Simply reserve three 45-minute blocks of time during your first week. Now schedule in week two. The ancient Chinese philosopher Lao-tzu said, "The journey of a thousand miles begins with one step." Congratulate yourself because you just made that first step.

It will also take a certain amount of time to reach your goal and to attain your version of a Hollywood body. If you have a body that resembles Camryn Manheim's, chances are you may never look like Calista Flockhart, but with effort and time you may indeed be able to attain a shape and size that could resemble those of Catherine Zeta-Jones. Such a transformation will not occur overnight, nor should it. The luxury of time is essential in not only changing the way your body looks but in changing your own self-image. I have coached many clients through the process of losing a great deal of body fat, and many who have shed in excess of 100 pounds of fat. Being comfortable in their new bodies took significant mental adjustment. With the luxury of time you will be mentally and emotionally equipped to accept the physical changes that are coming your way.

How long will *your* transformation take? It depends on what you are striving for.

If your goal is weight loss, you are in luck. The majority of my personal clients are celebrities who need to look their best in the shortest possible time. Weight loss generally boils down to a simple math problem, however, and you can only lose so much weight safely. Most experts agree that at best you can lose only 2 pounds of fat per week. To do this you really have to push yourself and be extremely active. It is much more reasonable to strive for 1 pound of fat loss per week. Although it may not seem dramatic, even a modest fat reduction of 1 pound per week becomes astounding when done consistently over time. If you can lose 1 pound of fat per week, you can be over 50 pounds lighter in one year, and over two years you could lose more than 100 pounds. Small, steady progress can add up to nearly miraculous results if you are patient and consistent.

Time Management

To get the greatest results and use your time wisely, it is essential that you begin using a scheduling aid. It doesn't matter what you use—it can be the electronic variety on your computer or hand-held, the paper variety in one of those leather binders, or an inexpensive spiral-bound calendar. I actually prefer the least expensive option, paper, and use a calendar that displays an entire week over two open pages, where each column is a day.

When the weekend comes, I strongly suggest that you set aside a few minutes on Saturday or Sunday to plan out your upcoming week. In your weekly schedule, you should block out time to do your grocery shopping and an afternoon or evening when you will prepare food for the coming week so that your food is ready to be warmed up when you need it.

Then schedule the times you will do your cardiovascular exercise and workouts. After you have made these entries you can pencil in regular appointments, chores, and meetings. When you are finished with these entries you can then take a "big picture" look at the week before you. You are prepared to see the holes in your schedule, so go about filling those time slots. Perhaps you would like to get in some additional activity—maybe you would like to play a round of golf, go for a bicycle ride, take a hike, or have a game of tennis. Remember, the more active you are, the more active you will become, and it is essential to push yourself.

With this organizing tool, you can easily see what you have to do on any given day, and clearly see that you could fit in even more. This simple tool will enable you to become more accountable to yourself, provide a disciplined system to support your new goals and priorities, give you greater control each day, and help you to become much more efficient and effective.

Before You Begin

Preparation is key. Before you begin, you will need some basic equipment. Make sure the listed items are available to you before you read chapter 6.

Your Hollywood Body Shopping List

- An exercise (therapy) ball.
- Two sets of dumbbells or one set with adjustable weights. Women should have a pair each of three-pound and five-pound dumbbells. Men should have a set of ten-pound and twenty-pound dumbbells.
- A set of ankle weights. You want the variety of ankle weights that can be adjusted. Women should have a pair that can accommodate 1 to 5 pounds. Men should have a pair that can accommodate 5 to 10 pounds.
- A fairly thick exercise mat (not a yoga mat).
- A heart-rate monitor (optional).
- A good pair of cross-training athletic shoes.
- Comfortable clothing that you can move in.
- A spiral-bound weekly schedule, day planner, or electronic scheduling aid.
- A good-quality multivitamin.
- A 32-ounce water bottle.

Starting the Program

The Hollywood body system begins with a two-week initiation. During this initiation you are going to reset your metabolism, establish a level of endurance, and increase your strength.

We'll start off slow and step up ever so slightly each day. By the end of the initiation, you will have trimmed inches, improved your physique, and achieved a fairly dramatic level of overall fitness and stamina.

The second portion of my program, which lasts four weeks, is where you will see the most dramatic physical changes. The four-week portion helps you get a Hollywood body for your personal body type.

There are three basic body types: the ectomorph, the meso-morph, and the endomorph. Each of these types faces unique challenges. For instance, an ectomorph has a hard time putting on weight, whether fat or muscle. Typically a thin, wiry type of build, this person can eat almost anything in any quantity and not gain an ounce. A mesomorph can generally put on muscle very easily. She or he has more of an athletic build: broad shoulders, wide back, and thick thigh muscles. This person has to watch what she eats and train very specifically or she will be adding fat onto her body. An endomorph only has to look at food and he gains weight—and not the right kind of weight. Some possible characteristics are narrow shoulders and a pear-shaped body.

I will help you identify which type best describes you, then we'll go to work on shaping and sculpting your problem areas. In six short weeks, you will have completely changed your shape and appearance—by the end of the month, your personal body type will be much more of a combination of the three. Then you can go to work on fine-tuning.

To complete your total-body makeover, I have created Final Cut, a revolutionary system to get you truly stunning results quickly, just like your favorite star. By the time you finish Final Cut, you too will be ready for the red carpet.

Secrets of the
Stars

Many people have been lured into buying a magazine because they saw a celebrity's photo on the cover and were pitched a how-to exercise story on how you can get that star's well-rounded butt. I know that I just can't resist those magazines, and I've even written my fair share of those articles. Do you really want to know how celebrities look so great? They work extremely hard to get those hard bodies. So let's cut to the chase—stars' bodies look like that because stars are dedicated, they watch what they eat, and they exercise intensely and often. You probably knew that, but what you may not know is that they really do have secrets to looking their best quickly. They do things in a very particular way, in a specific order, and there are special exercises to sculpt specific body parts to create an overall look. If they can do it, you can do it, and I'm here to help you.

Let's get very specific about what you most admire about the Hollywood body and how you want yours to look so that your efforts have a focus. The Hollywood bodies you most admire are the sum of many parts—that is, the backs of the arms, the derriere, the sculpted chest, the well-defined obliques, and the highly toned legs that all contribute to an overall look. You may notice one or two of these body parts as your favorite celebrity glides down the red carpet in a revealing designer outfit. Merely losing a certain amount of weight will not make you look like your favorite celebrity. However, if while losing that amount of weight you work to create proper muscular balance and definition, you will indeed look great. Throughout this book, I will teach you to take what you have and improve it into the best that it can be so that you achieve a total look that more closely resembles the body of your favorite star.

Spot Toning

Spot toning is truly the secret of attaining a Hollywood body. The next time you are watching your favorite celebrities walking down the red carpet or being interviewed on television, examine their various body parts. Focus on the small details and take in how and why certain areas of their bodies stand out. Look at the body parts containing large muscle groups, such as the legs, the back, the arms, the chest, and the abdomen. All of these muscle groups are the sum of many parts as well.

In examining the large muscle groups of the celebrity body, you will begin to see traits that you admire and may want to emulate. If you look closely enough, many things may begin to stick out. You will notice a certain symmetry that is dazzling. You will see balance between the upper and lower halves of the Hollywood body. Look closer and you will see that the right and left arms are the same size. The right and left legs are equally toned and muscular. The biceps are just about as large as the calves. As you begin, balance will be your primary focus.

It is not uncommon for most people to be out of balance. When we drive, we get out of the car by placing our left foot on the ground, and that leg supports our entire weight as we stand. As a consequence, the left thigh is generally stronger and larger than the right thigh. Also, we all have a dominant arm, and we use that arm most of the time. This dominant arm is probably stronger and larger than the other arm. This imbalance may extend to other body parts. Perhaps one of your shoulders is larger or higher, or one side of your back is more developed than the other. The muscles in your lower back may not be as strong or developed as your abdominal musculature. Aside from disrupting proper posture, these imbalances take away from looking fit.

Legs

Pay particular attention to your legs. When you are doing your sculpting exercises, you should strive to work your legs very hard. The harder you work them, the greater the results will be throughout the rest of your body. There should be a balance between the strength and size of the front and back of the thigh. Commonly, even with well-defined thighs, the rear of the thigh is not well developed. When the back of the thigh (hamstring) is bowed rather than flat, it will create a better line to accentuate the curvature of the buttocks, providing you with a more athletic and toned appearance.

There are some large muscles in the front of the thigh. Creating greater definition in this area will have fantastic payoffs. Achieving a line appearance down the side of the thigh provides the ultrafit, hard-body look that seems to be in vogue. For women especially, well-defined calves are the secret to looking your best and strutting your stuff. Other than being tortuous, high heels are designed to provide the calf with a certain flex, making it appear well defined and accentuating the muscle.

Buttocks

When you work on your gluteus maximus—your butt—you will need to develop the point of demarcation where the rear of the thigh meets the bottom of the buttocks. Strengthen the muscles on each cheek so that they have a rounded rather than flat appearance. Creating this kind of definition will help offset whatever effects gravity and genetics have had. The next priority, especially for men, is to develop the edges of the muscle, providing you with the "dimple" or hollow just outside the joint where your thigh and pelvic bone meet.

Back

The back is made up of a very large group of muscles that greatly accentuate your overall appearance. There are three celebrity secrets that can make the back truly stunning. First, there are the shoulder blades. You will be striving to achieve a well-defined musculature on the inside of each shoulder blade. Second, you will develop the trapezius (traps) muscles that look as if they sit on top of the actual shoulder blade. For both men and women, the development of these muscles makes the back sexier. Shaping these muscles will help the shoulder blades pull closer together. This will positively affect your posture, lifting your chest and rolling back your shoulders (the opposite of hunching your shoulders). Not only will you appear to be standing straighter and more lifted, but the musculature running down either side of the spine will be accentuated, providing you with an even more defined look. Third, and perhaps most important, you will strengthen the latissimus dorsi (lats) muscles. These winglike muscles begin in the center of your rib cage and reach up toward your armpits. Depending on your body type, you can develop these muscles to deemphasize a thick waist, create an hourglass figure, appear extremely athletic, or make your torso appear longer to emphasize your shoulders rather than your hips, or to appear extremely thin.

Chest

A developed chest can make men appear more virile and powerful, and for women it can be far more enhancing than plastic surgery. The strategy to achieve a Hollywood chest is remarkably similar for both men and women. Basically the chest muscle is shaped like a horseshoe. We will focus on developing and accentuating the outer edges of the horseshoe. It will then be easier to fill in the horseshoe and give the chest a more balanced look. You may notice that many box office idols have developed the upper portions of their pectoral muscles. Aside from defining the outer edge, this upper pectoral development is crucial. Female celebrities spend an even greater amount of time working this area. They concentrate on the upper pectoral area to enhance cleavage and make the collarbone more pronounced; however, they work the bottom half just as hard for lift, and they pay even closer attention to the inner edge of the pectoral muscle for breast separation as well as to accentuate the ribs connecting to the sternum.

Arms

The development and sculpting of the shoulder muscles can create a stunningly beautiful arm as well as proper posture. Read the next few sentences, then put this book down to determine if you have muscular imbalance. Simply stand up, extend your arms to the sides, release them, and let them fall. Let them bounce and come to a stop. Take notice of which way your palms are facing.

Chances are that your palms are facing behind you and your knuckles are facing forward (to some degree). If not, you represent 2 percent of the general population and probably do some kind of heavy manual labor such as working with a handsaw. The reason your knuckles are facing forward is that the rear portion of your shoulder is weaker than the front portion of the muscle. There are very few activities that will develop the rear portion of the shoulder, and it is precisely this section that is the coup de grace of the most stunning Hollywood bodies. Take a close look at your favorite female star wearing a sleeveless dress. Notice how there is a well-defined point of demarcation that separates the back of the shoulder and the tricep. For both men and women, that will be our focus for shoulder sculpting, as it is the most-prized secret of the stars.

Men and women have very different needs and goals for their arms. Women look to create a well-defined but decidedly feminine-looking arm, while most men shoot for size. For men, this area of the body is of singular importance. Men's biceps are a symbol of power and strength—an expression of manliness. While our intention will be to create a certain amount of bulk and definition, men should take a look at some celebrity biceps. This is a very simple muscle. It is connected to the skeletal system in just two places, and the only function of this muscle is to contract. Therefore, it becomes easy to have a very short little ball of a bicep.

While watching some celebrity arms, notice how long and relatively full their biceps are. While creating some bulk and a whole lot of definition in the biceps, one of our primary concerns is to develop an elongated bicep. But the biceps are only half of the arm. The main focus is to develop the two sides of the tricep muscle and strive for separation between them. Men should try to achieve a relative balance between the size of the biceps and triceps, and women should try to tone and cut the triceps. For women, the more defined the triceps—the more muscle separation you can achieve here—the better your arms will look.

Abdominals

The muscles that comprise the majority of the abdominal section of your body are like eight little boxes. In the gym, people refer to them as a six-pack, and if they are really defined, an eight-pack. Everyone has an eight-pack. Most of us, though, have subcutaneous fat (the fat underneath the skin) that prevents these muscles from being seen. If you can see muscle definition on the tummies of your favorite celebrities it is not because they have big abdominal muscles—it is because they have a very low body fat percentage.

The Hollywood Body Triangle

When the three elements of the Hollywood body system are put together into a comprehensive program, your results are guaranteed. With Hollywood nutrition, you will be feeding lean muscle and burning fat. With Hollywood heart, you will improve your circulation, strengthen your heart, increase your endurance, become more physically fit, and most important, you will be using stored fat to fuel your activity. With Hollywood sculpt, you will be reshaping each muscle from its deepest point. When all three sides of this training triangle are in place, nothing can prevent you from attaining a Hollywood body.

By bringing all three sides of the training triangle together, you create a momentum. Your nutritional program supports your cardiovascular program. Your sculpting program supports your cardiovascular activity and your diet. As each day passes, the three elements of your transformation take a firmer hold. You begin feeling the changes and seeing the changes when you look in the mirror. When your aerobic training, weight training, and diet are all working to complement one another, something magical happens. You begin coasting downhill. You do not have to work as hard, but your transformation unfolds rapidly. Changes occur faster, dramatically affecting the way you look and feel.

No matter what level of exercise you currently enjoy, whether you are just beginning or have practiced these three disciplines all your life, you should carefully read the next three chapters. If you are just beginning, use this information as if it were a one-on-one session with your personal trainer. You will learn the philosophy and the scientific principles that are the basis for your transformation. If you have been exercising for years, attempt to rethink your currently held convictions. You will pick up at least a few precious gems that will take your level of fitness to heights previously unknown to you.

Hollywood Nutrition Principles

3

Dieting has become an American obsession. Diet and nutrition are *the* most talked about topics in our popular culture. You cannot walk through a grocery store, turn on the TV, listen to the radio, or open your e-mail without being bombarded with the latest fad diet that promises a thinner you.

Weight is an issue for almost everyone. Some of us really have to watch every bite that we eat; with much suffering and sacrifice, we are able to lose a little. Some of us have tried every diet, but nothing works. There are also people at the other extreme—who have to try very hard to maintain their weight. Too much work or running around, and they are dropping weight like nobody's business. For them, gaining weight would be a dream come true. Most of us are somewhere between these two extremes. You must understand both ends of the spectrum to figure out what will work best for you.

Body Fat

Your goal is to eliminate body fat. You will need the proper method to determine if your program is working. Your scale does not provide a clear picture of what is happening to your body. Your weight on the scale is only a small factor of this total picture. Before you begin, take measurements of your waist, hips, chest, each bicep, and thigh. This will provide valuable information to not only mark your progress but also to determine and concentrate your efforts.

While the easiest method to determine results will be to monitor how your clothes are fitting, most of us need a more telling measurement. In addition to taking measurements of various body parts, I recommend you determine your body fat percentage. This measurement will be your new guide and key indicator of your progress. It will provide you with a clear picture of what percentage of your total body weight is made up of fat and what percentage is made up of water, hair, bone, and lean muscle mass. Your goal is to create more bone and muscular density and reduce the percentage of fat.

How to Measure Your Body Fat

There are many ways to measure your body fat, such as hydrostatic weighing and bioimpedance, and there is a cost associated with taking these measurements. While going into a local gym and having a trained professional take a few measurements with skinfold calipers might cost $15, some other (and very accurate) methods might cost thousands. In truth, you can get a fairly good idea of your own body fat percentage in the privacy of your own home, at absolutely no cost. You will need a scale, a tape measure (a new cloth or metal tape is preferable), a calculator, and perhaps an assistant.

BODY FAT FORMULA FOR WOMEN

1. Step on the scale and weigh yourself.
   Your body weight _____ × 0.732 + 8.987 = _____

2. Measure your wrist at the fullest point.
   Your wrist measurement _____ ÷ 3.140 = _____

3. Measure your waist at your navel.

   Your waist measurement _____ × 0.157 = _____

4. Measure your hips at the fullest point.

   Your hip measurement _____ × 0.249 = _____

5. Measure your forearm at the fullest point.

   Your forearm measurement _____ × 0.434 = _____

Now calculate your body fat. On your calculator:

   Add the totals for 1 and 2.

   Subtract the total for 3.

   Subtract the total for 4.

   Add the total for 5.

This number is your lean body mass (muscle, bones, organs, hair, etc.).

   Subtract your lean body mass from your total weight

   Total body weight _____ – lean body mass _____ = _____

This number is the weight of your body fat.

   Body fat weight _____ × 100 = _____ ÷ Total body weight = _____

This number is your body fat percentage.

BODY FAT FORMULA FOR MEN

1. Step on the scale and weigh yourself.

   Your body weight _____ × 1.082 + 94.42 = _____

2. Measure your waist.

   Your waist measurement _____ × 4.15 = _____

Now calculate your body fat. On your calculator:

   Subtract the total for 2 from the total for 1.

   Measurement 1 _____ – Measurement 2 = _____

This number is your lean body mass.

Subtract your lean body mass from your total weight.

Total body weight _____ – lean body mass _____ = _____

This number is the weight of your body fat.

Body fat weight ____ × 100 = ____ ÷ Total body weight = _____

This number is your body fat percentage.

Body Fat Basics

There are some basic rules about body fat. It is stored within fat cells. You are born with a certain number of those fat cells, which you essentially inherited from your ancestors. Those with ancestors from Northern Europe inherit more fat cells than those who are descended from people nearer to the equator. Until the end of puberty, you can grow even more fat cells. After puberty, you will not grow any more fat cells, but the cells you have will either grow or shrink. Any given fat cell can grow to be as large as your head or shrink so small that several dozen could fit on the head of a pin.

You have and need a small percentage of fat. If you pinch the skin on the top of your hand (as opposed to your love handles or "saddle bags") you can clearly see what "enough" means. For women, this minimal amount is 12 to 15 percent of your total body weight; for men, it is about 5 percent. Very fit and highly trained people can achieve these low percentages, but it is much more reasonable for women to be closer to the 20 percent range. Dip far below this and you might experience a loss of menstrual cycle, hair loss, and/or a loss of bone density. Men can strive for a healthy 12 to 14 percent.

Body fat exists for your survival and should be thought of much like a reserve tank of fuel. It prevents starvation, and this starvation protection mechanism is hardwired into your system. To eliminate body fat, you need to outthink your natural starvation protection mechanism.

Outthink Your Body

Your starvation protection mechanism is a primal system to ensure your survival. This system regulates what and how much energy to release to maintain your most basic bodily functions. The only tool this complex system uses is the regulation of body fat. In times of extreme hardship when there are prolonged periods without food, your body's starvation protection mechanism works overtime—it stores almost every nutrient you eat within fat cells for later use. It then conserves all the energy it can and uses the barest minimum to keep your heart beating and your lungs breathing.

This primal survival system has no idea that it is living in the twenty-first century. It does not know that food is as close as the nearest drive-thru window and that going without food does not equate to starvation. When you go for long periods without food, all this primal system knows is that you are not being taken care of. Your body equates not eating regularly with *danger*. When it experiences danger, it stores all it can within fat cells and releases very little of what is held in those cells.

If you are not eating enough food for an extended period of time, something even more significant will occur. Your body needs energy, and you require energy to perform any activity. So when the starvation protection mechanism senses danger, it goes into survival mode and shuts down fat cells. If and when you do eat, most of these nutrients get stored within fat cells. Aside from fueling enough energy for heart and lung functions, this mechanism will not let any fat out of these cells. But you still need to walk from here to there or do whatever you have to do to get some food. That energy needs to come from someplace. Your body can easily consume body tissue to get these essential nutrients to fuel your activity. In the body's starvation mode, muscle tissue, organ tissue, and brain tissue are literally cannibalized to provide you with the fuel you need.

When most people go on a diet, they do not lose fat; they lose *random weight*. Approximately one-third of your weight on the scale is water, and most diets and diet products are simply diuretics. If you see products that say you can lose 10 pounds in 48 hours, this kind of water weight is exactly what you will lose. Diet centers and fad diets, however, will reduce your food (caloric) intake, and will do so to such a drastic extent that your body will think it is starving. If the diet is extreme—and most are—you will step on the scale and see that you have lost weight. But that weight loss will be water, muscle, and bone, but very little if any fat loss.

When you can outsmart your natural fat storage system, you can naturally and effectively eliminate stored fat. To do this, you need to eat regularly and often. Most people make two serious mistakes: they wait too long to eat, activating the starvation alarm, or they eat too much, activating the fat storage system. This results in the body storing almost all of what we eat as body fat because it fears starvation.

To reduce fat, your starvation protection device needs to be lulled into a sense of security. This is accomplished by eating a small snack-size meal every $2^{1}/_{2}$ to 3 hours at approximately the same times every day. When this becomes a regular pattern—after two weeks or so—your body will begin to trust that it does not have to be on alert because there are no danger signs of shortage or starvation. When the starvation protection device relaxes sufficiently, it will begin releasing the nutrients stored within your fat cells, since they are no longer needed to ensure your survival.

Eating small snack-size meals at regular intervals is key, but to attain the Hollywood body in the shortest amount of time, you must choose *what* to eat carefully and thoughtfully.

Combining Proteins and Carbohydrates

During the digestive process, the molecular structure of food is broken down into smaller and smaller bits until these bits are small enough to pass through the intestinal wall and are released into the bloodstream. Once set free into the bloodstream, they can be used by the parts of the body that need them most. Your body ultimately derives amino acids from eating protein. Amino acids feed lean muscle. The less fatty the protein, the more efficiently your lean muscle can utilize the amino acids.

When carbohydrates are digested, they are ultimately broken down into sugar or glucose. You need a certain amount of glucose to keep the body functioning properly, but when there is too much glucose in the bloodstream, it will cause a hormone called insulin to be secreted. Insulin has one job: to take out all the extra glucose in the bloodstream and store it within the fat cells just in case it is needed in the future. Once nutrients are stored away in fat cells the body is very reluctant to part with what it has stored. It is therefore your primary objective not to flood the bloodstream with too much glucose.

When choosing a carbohydrate, you will want to eat something that takes a long period of time to break apart in the digestive process, and you will find these foods listed in this chapter as primary carbohydrate selections. Because the molecular chains of these particular carbohydrates are difficult to break apart, glucose is released into the bloodstream slowly over a longer period of time. The more difficulty the body has in breaking apart the molecular chain of the carbohydrate, the higher the carbohydrate will appear on the list.

I am certain you know what fat is. Fat is butter, oil, lard—the stuff that hangs over your belt, the stuff you want less of. Fat is essential for the body. However, almost every living organism on the planet contains some fat, so it is not necessary to add any extra fat to your food. When cooking, you should try to eliminate most, if not all, of the fat you can. Unfortunately, fat does add to the taste of food, so if you are going to add it, add it by the drop and not by the spoonful or cupful.

Portion Size

For any given meal, first decide which source of protein you will be eating, then determine the carbohydrate choice and corresponding portion size. If you want to rid yourself of fat, the portion size of your protein should be approximately the size of your palm. If you want to maintain your present weight, your protein portion should be the size of your palm extended to first joint of your fingers. If you would like to gain muscle mass, your protein portion should be the size of your hand. You will find a food list in this chapter that outlines which protein choices are best. Good proteins are found in protein powder, egg whites, most fish, skinless chicken breast, and turkey breast. These proteins have little inherent fat and are absorbed most effectively by your body's digestive system.

Secondary protein choices should be cut or very sparingly selected in your nutritional program. They include choice cuts of beef that are highly marbled, pork products, sausages, processed meats, cold cuts, duck, goose, lamb, and cheese. All of these secondary choices contain a higher proportion of fat and are not absorbed as effectively by the digestive system.

After your two-week initiation phase (described in chapter 6), you will combine your foods in a specific manner. Based on your choice of protein, you will then determine which carbohydrate and how much of that carbohydrate you should have. For instance, if you choose to eat one item from the list of primary protein selections, you can have twice that amount from the list of primary carbohydrate selections or the exact same-size portion of secondary carbohydrate selections. If you are eating a skinless chicken breast, you can have twice the amount of steamed cauliflower (a 1:2 ratio), or the same-size portion of rice, potato, bread, or pasta (a 1:1 ratio). If you choose to eat a secondary source of protein, you can have the same amount of a good carbohydrate or half that amount of a secondary carbohydrate. If you choose to eat a fatty protein such as beef pot roast, you can eat that same portion size of steamed vegetables or half the portion size of your protein in pasta. In addition, there are a number of free foods that do not count toward the equation, and you may have as much of them as you like if you are still hungry.

PRIMARY PROTEIN SELECTIONS

Chicken breast (not processed)

Cottage cheese (low- or nonfat)

Egg substitutes

Egg whites

Fat-free cheese

Fish (any)

Lean ground beef (15 percent fat or lower)

Mock chicken or mock duck

Protein powder (whey)

Shellfish (any)

Soy burger

Soy hot dog

Soy sausage

Tempeh

Tofu

Turkey breast (not processed)

All others = secondary protein selection, which includes higher-fat red meats and poultry

PRIMARY CARBOHYDRATE SELECTIONS

Vegetables

Artichokes	Chickpeas	Mushrooms
Asparagus	Dried beans (any)	Navy beans
Bok choy	Eggplant	Pinto beans
Broccoli	Green beans	Red beans
Brussels sprouts	Kale	Soy beans
Butter beans	Kidney beans	Spinach
Cabbage	Lentils	Squash
Cauliflower	Lima beans	Zucchini

Starches

Brown rice	Egg noodles

Fruits

Apples	Grapefruit	Plums
Apricots (dried)	Oranges	Prunes
Berries (all)	Peaches	Tomatoes
Cherries	Pears	

Dairy

Nonfat yogurt with fruit and sugar substitute	Nonfat plain yogurt with sugar substitute	Nonfat fruit-flavored yogurt with sugar

SECONDARY CARBOHYDRATE SELECTIONS

Starches and Carbohydrates

Bread (all)	Most rice	Most pasta
Potatoes (all)	Most cereals	

Vegetables

Beets	Corn	Pumpkin
Carrots	Peas	

Fruits

Applesauce	Figs	Papaya
Apricots	Grapes	Pineapple
Bananas	Kiwi	Raisins
Cantaloupe	Honeydew	Watermelon
Cranberries	Kumquats	
Dates	Mango	

FREE FOODS

Celery	Lettuce (iceberg, romaine, butter lettuce, endive, radicchio)	Salsa
Cucumber		Sugar-free ice tea
Crystal Light		Sugar-free instant cocoa
Garlic	Lime juice	Sugar-free Jell-O
Jicama	Mustard	Sugar-free popsicles
Kohlrabi	Peppers	Sugar-free sodas
Lemon juice	Radishes	Vinegar

There are a number of ways that you can play with the 1:1/1:2 model. If you choose an excellent protein source and are craving a piece of bread, you can fit it into your meal in the following way: Look at the portion of protein on your plate. Divide that surface area in half. That will be the portion of your bread. You can have the same-size portion of primary carbohydrates, and you will have completed the 1:2 meal. I know it is really more like the 1:1$\frac{1}{2}$ meal, but you got the bread and you didn't make yourself crazy. Still hungry? A small tossed salad is a free food; it does not count and is not part of the equation unless you have croutons or add a dressing other than vinegar, lemon, or a little salsa. So you might have a chicken breast, some vegetables, a little bread, and a salad. That is a really nice meal, and you wouldn't feel like you were suffering if you did this five times a day. If you choose a secondary protein, simply have the same-size portion of primary carbohydrates or half that protein portion size of a secondary carbohydrate choice. Easy, right?

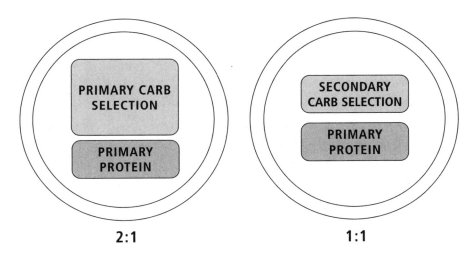

Reminders, Hints, and Tricks

To recap, you should have at least five small meals per day, eating about every three hours. Have breakfast, lunch, and dinner, and between these main meals have a snack consisting of a protein bar or shake, nonfat cottage cheese and fruit, or even a chicken breast with some raw or lightly steamed vegetables. Choose your protein first, then the appropriate carbohydrate choice.

If you go out to eat, immediately order a tossed salad with dressing on the side. The point is to avoid the bread that will be placed on the table. People dig into this bread as a matter of habit without fully realizing the amount of carbohydrates they are ingesting. I attempt to refrain from alcohol, but if you really need a glass of wine or a mixed drink, go ahead. If you have one drink—and I do mean *one* glass—this will count as your carbohydrate for the meal. Your meal might consist of a large dinner salad with lemon, a nice cut of beef or chicken breast, and a glass of wine.

Occasionally you will have cravings. A great trick is to brush your teeth right after meals. It has been reported that this curbs the desire for desserts. You can also curb cravings by choosing one meal each week where you can eat whatever you like. If you have seven or eight of these meals per week, chances are you will not see any results. This program takes some discipline, but it will become second nature after only a couple of weeks. Give yourself the gift of eating properly for those two weeks.

You should have a minimum of eight glasses of water a day. The body operates much better when it is hydrated. You are made up of almost two-thirds water, so it makes sense that you need to replenish as much as possible. Water is one of the best ways to rid yourself of fat, and to feel full even if you are eating less food. Start with eight glasses a day and work your way up to more. Try drinking a glass before and after each meal.

Keep a journal. If you have a day planner or an electronic wizard, record what you ate, when you ate, and how many glasses of water you drank during the day. This practice will help you in your discipline. For some reason, when people begin to keep track of what they eat, they are better able to stick with their program.

Plan ahead. Make certain that you have enough groceries on hand so that you do not order a pizza or go to the hamburger drive-thru out of desperation. Know what you are going to be eating. Plan your meals each day. If you work in an office, keep food in the fridge. Have some protein bars in your desk. Know which restaurants in your area serve or deliver the kind of food that you need. Above all, this way of eating should not involve depriving yourself and should fit into your life reasonably.

And remember—never eat less than 1,000 calories per day or

your body will shift into starvation mode, making it impossible to shed body fat.

As you'll see, the Hollywood nutrition portion of the Hollywood body plan begins with a two-week initiation into a new way of eating. Like high-protein plans, you will eliminate all simple carbohydrates during this phase, reduce saturated fats, eat many greens and vegetables, and limit your intake of caffeine. During these two weeks, you will break unhealthy patterns, short-circuit your food cravings or food addictions, and effectively reset your metabolism.

4

Hollywood Heart
Principles

The great catalyst for the Hollywood body system and the most addictive and self-gratifying element of this program is without question cardiovascular activity. It will give you immediate results: feelings of well-being, reduction of stress levels, increased energy, clarity of thought, and an increased ability to focus and to relax more fully.

In the long term, my prescription for cardiovascular activity will enable you to reach your maximum heart health, and you will reduce the likelihood of diseases such as diabetes, heart attack, stroke, and even cancer. While you achieve these very significant gains in overall health and reduce the risk of many diseases, you will also improve the way you look. Within a week or two, you will notice improvements in the quality of your skin and hair. But the most significant improvement in your appearance will be rapid fat reduction.

The Hollywood heart principles eliminate excess body fat and increase your level of fitness, endurance, and overall health. Your physical transformation can take place only with the support of a sound nutritional program coupled with regular cardiovascular activity. You will be given guidelines so that you can create the program that best suits your needs. This personalized program will bring you toward your goal quickly, safely, and efficiently.

Why Should I Exercise?

You simply have to do cardiovascular exercise. Your life depends on it. Ongoing studies provide irrefutable evidence that you must exercise regularly in order to stay healthy.

According to the Centers for Disease Control and the Department of Health and Human Services, inactivity leads to weight gain. Being overweight and inactive are the causative factors in more than 3 million deaths per year. These reputable sources have projected that overweight and inactivity will soon surpass tobacco-related illnesses as the number one killer in the United States.

You do not need to run hundreds of miles every week. The Surgeon General recommends exercising at least one hour each day, but at minimum you need to exercise at least three times per week. If you do, looking great will be the least of what you get.

The true importance of aerobic or cardiovascular activity in the Hollywood body system is to speed your metabolism, eliminate body fat, and attain a leaner physique. The fitter you become, the more calories your body will burn when you are at rest. A better-trained individual will burn 20 percent more calories at rest than a sedentary person. As you become more and more fit, it will not take as much effort to maintain the results you achieve.

There are many attributes and even more long-term health benefits associated with regular cardiovascular exercise. Along with possibly decreasing your appetite, exercising within your ideal target range allows for greater caloric intake without gaining fat. Cardiovascular exercise has been scientifically proven to strengthen your skeletal system, creating bone density and combating osteoporosis. This form of exercise is most often a part of the treatment for people with a history of diabetes, heart attack, high blood pressure, and/or high cholesterol. In addition to reducing the risk of coronary artery disease, regular cardiovascular exercise helps those suffering from arthritis. Perhaps the greatest benefit is that aerobically fit people deal with stress much more effectively; stress might be the number one health risk in our society.

For most people, the point is to get your body hot—literally and figuratively. This means warming your muscles up, supercharging your metabolism to burn off excess calories, and elevating your heart rate to a certain level for a specific period of time to melt the fat off your body. When you can do this regularly and consistently, you will call upon stored fat to fuel your activity. You will burn up your caloric intake. And soon you will look absolutely hot.

Aerobic and Anaerobic Exercise

When you exercise, you burn calories to fuel your activity. The point is to burn those calories off in the most efficient manner possible. There are two levels of exercise and consequently two ways that you can burn off calories: *anaerobic* and *aerobic*. Both of these terms refer to the manner in which the calorie is utilized or burned by your body. When you exercise and elevate your heart rate significantly, blood passes through the muscles being worked. To fuel that activity, the muscle extracts its fuel from the blood cell. When you are exercising at 50 to 70 percent of your maximum heart rate, glucose is extracted from the blood cell. At this level of exercise, you are in an aerobic state. When your heart rate reaches 85 percent of its maximum, there is so much blood pumping through your system that your body does not have enough time to process it all. To get around this dilemma, it simply burns the cell wall, or mitochondria, to fuel the activity. When this occurs, you are in an anaerobic state.

You can exercise at an aerobic level for a very long time. When you reach an anaerobic level, however, you can sustain it for only about 10 seconds before you either have to slow down or stop. If you are running a 100-yard dash, you might be in an aerobic state for the first seven seconds of the race. If you really kick it into high gear and push yourself to your physical limit, you will achieve an anaerobic state for only the last three seconds of the race. When you are in an anaerobic state, you are truly exhausting the energy supply because you are burning through the blood cells at such a rapid rate. The mitochondria cannot provide the muscles with the pure energy they need to keep going. After reaching the anaerobic state for a maximum duration of 5 to 10 seconds, the body shuts down, and you are forced to either slow down or stop altogether. You may have seen examples of this if you have ever watched Olympic runners. Some of the participants may peak too early in the race, and at the end of the race they appear to be slowing down rather than accelerating toward the finish line.

Another example is weight lifting. As you will soon experience, you will be asking yourself to perform three sets of a specific weight-lifting exercise. Each of these sets is made up of several repetitions. You will be at an aerobic level for the great majority of the set, but during the last three or four repetitions, you will feel fatigued. You will have to struggle to push the weight until you reach a point of muscular failure and are no longer physically able to perform another repetition. You will have reached the anaerobic phase of the exercise, and your body will force you to stop.

With Hollywood heart principles, you will consciously manipulate the aerobic and anaerobic states to meet your goals. The program is very simple to follow and is easy to incorporate into your lifestyle. During your workout, you will begin with five minutes of aerobics to warm up the muscles in your body. By stretching between resistance exercises, you will remain in an aerobic state. To end your workout, you will perform at least 25 minutes of the aerobic activity of your own choosing. You will consciously reach anaerobic levels several times during each session.

Getting Aerobic

To reach an aerobic level, you need to elevate your heart rate. Your body will burn calories most efficiently when your heart rate is between 60 and 80 percent of its maximum rate. You may want a calculator to determine these numbers, and you should write these numbers down so that you can refer to them later.

The medical establishment has determined that the human heart cannot safely beat more than 220 times per minute. Your own maximum heart rate is considerably lower. To determine your maximum heart rate, simply subtract your age from 220. For instance, if you are 40 years old, your maximum heart rate is 180 (220 − 40 = 180).

This number will be your personal ceiling. You *never* want to reach this number. When you are performing the cardiovascular program, you will want to maintain your heart rate in the 60 to 70 percent range for the majority of your session. So let's determine what that means in terms of your personal target area. Using our example of the person who is 40 years old, he or she should multiply 180×0.60, then multiply 180×0.80. The ideal aerobic level for a 40-year-old is when the heart beats between 108 and 144 times per minute.

Do one last calculation to determine where you reach your anaerobic state. You will consciously enter this range for a brief period of time to achieve a desired result. The anaerobic state is reached when you achieve 90 percent of your maximum heart rate. Using the 40-year-old as an example, the number is determined by multiplying the maximum heart rate of 180 by 0.90 ($180 \times 0.90 = 162$). When the person's heart rate reaches 162 beats per minute, he or she will only be able to sustain that activity for a maximum of ten seconds, then will either have to slow way down or stop altogether.

Monitoring Your Heart Rate

Now that you have calculated your ideal heart rates, you need to know how to find your pulse. There are three methods to determine how many times per minute your heart is beating. Two of these methods can be done manually with the aid of a clock or a stopwatch, and the other uses a small machine. You can take your own pulse on two points of the body: the wrist and the neck. Finding these spots takes a little practice, but after you have identified them and become familiar with them, they will prove to be fairly decent indicators of your heart rate.

The point on the wrist is sometimes easier to find. Locate the point at which your forearm meets your hand. Place your pointing and middle fingers in the middle of that area. (Never use your thumb as this finger has its own pulse.) You will feel a tendon or even several tendons in your wrist. Move your fingers slowly to the inside portion of your wrist until you can find the pulse at its strongest point.

You can also accurately measure your pulse on the neck at the carotid artery. To find this artery, locate the point where the front of your neck muscles meets your throat. Move your fingers slowly up the inside neck muscles until you find the point at which the pulse is the strongest.

With your fingers on either your wrist or your neck, look at a clock that has a second hand or at a stopwatch. Count the number of heartbeats for 15 seconds. Multiply that number by 4, and you have successfully determined your heart rate. If this gets too complicated or cumbersome, there is a third option.

There are a number of heart monitors on the market. I prefer these devices over taking my own pulse since they are more accurate and less of a hassle. These heart monitors are small and inconspicuous; they are usually attached to a belt or an elastic strap. The belt is placed around your chest. The monitor relays information to a watch worn on your wrist. While you are exercising, you only have to look at your wristwatch to check your heart rate.

The reason for monitoring our heart rate is threefold. First, studies have proven that people who exercise at 60 to 70 percent of their maximum heart rate level are much more likely to exercise regularly. If you have ever attempted regular exercise and have stopped for no apparent reason, you may have been exercising at a rate that your body could not sustain. It is far more taxing for your body to operate at 85 percent of your maximum. If you do so over an extended period of time, you may get burned out and quit exercising altogether. Second, you want to make this program time-efficient and get the greatest results in the quickest possible manner. Third, exercising at 60 percent to 70 percent of your maximum heart rate is the exact level at which the body burns fat most efficiently.

How Long Should I Exercise?

When you are exercising aerobically, you need to keep your heart rate in the 60 to 70 percent range for at least 25 minutes to have the desired results. When you are in your ideal aerobic range for this length of time, you will burn calories at the most efficient rate possible. For the first ten minutes or so, the body will use the glucose within the blood stream to fuel the motion—that is, you will be expending the excess calories you have eaten. For the next 15 minutes, your bloodstream will not be able to provide your body with all its needed fuel, so it will have to call upon its reserve tank, or stored fat, to provide the necessary energy. In these all-important 15 minutes, you will be fueling half of your activity with glucose that is still in the bloodstream. The other half of the expended calories will be derived from burning up fat stored underneath your skin.

If you can stay nearer to 70 percent of your maximum heart rate throughout your workout, you can call upon an even greater percentage of stored fat. If your goal is to rid yourself of body fat more quickly, you may want to devote more time to your cardiovascular workout. You could exercise aerobically for several hours, but the truth is that after 60 minutes or so, you will have maximized your workout. My recommendation is to do at least 25 minutes of cardiovascular exercise and no more than one hour, unless you are consciously performing extra aerobic activity to achieve a specific fitness goal.

How Often Should I Exercise?

You should perform this cardiovascular workout at least three times per week and can safely do it as many as six days per week. As with all forms of exercise, you must take at least one day off per week to let the body rest, heal, and recuperate. It is best to space out the days of your cardiovascular exercise to get the greatest results. Instead of performing your workouts on three consecutive days and resting for four, space the workouts evenly throughout the week. You will boost your metabolism, burn calories more efficiently, and ultimately have greater success.

Vary It

The single most vital ingredient to maximizing your cardiovascular workout is to vary it. The body is very reluctant to rid itself of body fat, and you must outthink it consistently. The body is resilient and will conserve its fuel whenever it can, so you must trick it. If you do the exact same cardiovascular exercise each and every time you work out, after only a short while the body will give up less and less stored fat.

If you run on a treadmill, you may want to increase or decrease the incline level every other time you work out. If you jog around a track, instead of running around the track at the exact same pace, you may want to do bursts to elevate the heart rate to 85 percent, then bring it back down to the ideal range, then vary the length of those bursts. Better yet, you may want to get off the track and jog through different areas of your neighborhood, each day finding different terrain. Many of the machines I will talk about have different courses that simulate this exact principle. You should make a note of which course you did last and be certain to change it for the next workout. You may choose to perform completely different exercises on different days. By employing some or all of these strategies, you will keep your body in a state of surprise. In this way, you can keep your body guessing and always demand the maximum results for your efforts.

By varying your routine, and always increasing and decreasing the level of difficulty while you exercise, you push yourself to become more physically fit. As you become more fit, your aerobic ceiling will increase. This is what you are striving for. Instead of becoming fatigued when you exercise at 60 percent of your maximum heart rate, you may have to increase to 70 or 80 percent as you grow stronger. It will take more effort to shift into an anaerobic gear.

You can increase your performance envelope by practicing terrain variance. If you walk or even jog on a hilly terrain or have the computerized resistance level on the treadmill set to vary the incline level, there will be times when you achieve an anaerobic level of exercise. As you near the top of the hill, your body is working harder. As a result, your heart rate increases to a point at which you may reach an anaerobic level. Typically, the signals that you have reached this anaerobic stage will include a shortness of breath, lactic acid buildup, and the onset of rapid fatigue. When you can facilitate brief encounters with the anaerobic stage and come back into your target area of 60 to 70 percent, you will successfully improve your physical condition, eliminate much of the glucose in the bloodstream, and consequently burn a greater number of calories from stored fat as you return to your targeted aerobic range.

Just Do It!

There are many different ways to achieve a healthy cardiovascular level, and there are no excuses for avoiding this important element of your transformation. If you have a tendency to avoid cardiovascular exercise like the plague, I ask you to recommit yourself to the process. Challenge and push yourself. Promise yourself that you will do ten minutes. After those first ten minutes are up, you are less likely to give up on yourself. During those first minutes, try to visualize your goal. Whatever your goal, your transformation depends heavily on doing your cardiovascular workout. You have a vast array of options, and there is no reason that you should ever become bored by your choices.

Again, the only thing that matters is that you do something to elevate your heart rate for at least 25 minutes. I prefer individual activities so that I do not have the excuse of "my partner didn't show up" for not doing my aerobics. I also prefer to do my aerobic workout immediately after I finish strength training. That is just my personal preference, but when you use the Hollywood sculpt program to tone your musculature, you will be lifting weights. There will be an increased amount of lactic acid in your body after weight lifting, and completing the cardiovascular portion after your toning session may prevent a great deal of soreness.

Choose whatever activity you enjoy. If you like to ride your mountain bike, row in a skull, or play handball, go for it. If you like to swim, play tennis, or swing dance, by all means do it. The point is to be active. If you do not know what you enjoy, try several things.

To Begin, Walk

If you are just beginning to exercise and have not been physically active for a while, begin by walking. It is actually a very efficient and effective method to increase your fitness level and achieve your goals.

The simpler you can make this process, the better. If you can't get to a gym to use an elliptical trainer, does that mean you cannot get in your cardiovascular exercise? If your tennis partner cancels, is that your excuse to skip your workout? No excuses here. If all you have to do is tie your sneakers and walk out the door, you eliminate any barriers that may prevent you from reaching your goal. If the weather does not permit you to walk outdoors, do it indoors. You may live or work in a high-rise building and choose to walk up and down the stairs. At almost every mall in the country, dozens of people gather before the stores open to get in their walk. In many areas there are hockey rinks, indoor sporting arenas, school gyms, and public buildings that could provide a venue for your cardiovascular workout. If you are healthy and mobile, there are no excuses. I have been shocked to see the numbers of people jogging along the rivers in Boston, New York City, and Philadelphia during torrential rains, and I have been awestruck by people speed-walking along the lakes in downtown Minneapolis, Chicago, Buffalo, and Detroit during snowstorms. While some people might think these exercisers are nuts, you will soon know why they do it. It makes you feel so good, you can't imagine *not* doing it.

If you walk to get in your cardiovascular exercise, you can achieve amazing results. If you walk one mile, you will probably burn about 100 calories. If you jogged that same mile, you would burn approximately 110 calories. There is really not much of a difference. I have seen people lose up to 120 pounds by walking. All you need to do is raise your heart rate to the target range for at least 25 minutes.

If you choose to walk, it is not the kind of walking you do as you window shop. You must walk at a brisk pace with energetic motion in your arms. If you'd like, you can bring a set of 2-pound dumbbells (to avoid injury, *never* use ankle weights) on your walk to increase the intensity of your workout. Intensity is the key.

Assuming you are just beginning, elevate your heart rate level to

60 percent of your max and maintain this level for at least 25 minutes. After you are able to achieve this, do not increase the duration of your walk, but increase the intensity. When you are able to achieve 60 percent of your maximum heart rate for 25 consecutive minutes, you are ready for the entire Hollywood workout.

5

Hollywood Sculpt Principles

The Strategy

Superstar Hollywood bodies look very different today than they did in the 1970s, the 1980s, or even the 1990s. Today the look is all about lean and chiseled. The days of the Incredible Hulk and Conan the Barbarian have been replaced by the Tobey Maguire–type superhero. Where musclemen once ruled, there are now the Brad Pitt and George Clooney–esque bodies that feature elongated but highly toned musculature. Women now have many Hollywood role models to look to for inspiration. Star bodies are no longer demure stick figures but come in all shapes and sizes. Without question, most of these Hollywood bodies have much in common, and both male and female prototypes rely on leanness as well as muscle tone and definition to accentuate their star power. How do these Hollywood bodies look their best? They do it through weight training.

After your nutritional and cardiovascular programs are in place, real and dramatic change can occur. In essence, your nutritional and cardiovascular programs complement and aid each other in eliminating stored fat. With this combination, the former you will begin to melt away and will soon reveal the new exterior you will work so diligently to create. The real transformation, however, occurs with strengthening, toning, and sculpting the muscles underneath that layer of body fat. Hollywood sculpt principles are part of a revolutionary program that shapes, sculpts, and rebuilds each muscle from its deepest point so that you can experience a total and complete physical transformation. By also using Hollywood nutrition and Hollywood heart principles, you will reduce your body fat and enable the shell of the old you to melt into the *new you*.

Everyone has a part of their body they are not comfortable with. Even the fittest and most beautiful celebrities wish they could improve some part of their physique. Why should you be any different? I will teach you the secrets of the stars and help you create a look that you are happy with. There are many secrets to making each muscle group look the best that it can be and reshaping the muscle to complement and accentuate the whole package. All you have to do is follow the directions and sweat a little, and you will soon look the way you want to look.

Body Symmetry

I have encouraged you to take the measurements of various body parts. These measurements are key. Not only will they allow you to track progress, but they will also focus your work. Nature loves nothing more than symmetry, and when the body and all of its parts strike a balance, the whole is more aesthetically appealing.

The first objective is to create a symmetric balance. You should strive to have each arm and each leg the same size, and work toward your calves being the same size as your biceps. For each body part and muscle group, there is a strategy to make it look its best.

Toning and Shaping

Resistance training, commonly known as weight training, is one of the most misunderstood and maligned forms of exercise. Given the many misconceptions surrounding weight training, fear often replaces reason for would-be enthusiasts. Many people look at weight training with skepticism. Many women are hesitant to exercise with weights for fear that they will get bulky or look manly. The elderly fear that weight training will somehow injure them. Many people who are overweight fear that weight training will only make them bigger. Nothing could be farther from the truth. For all shapes and sizes, weight training is the most effective means to create lean muscle mass and positively change appearance.

Lean muscle mass is the greatest asset you can have. By increasing lean muscle mass, you automatically reduce the percentage of fat you are carrying around. Lean muscle mass burns more calories than fat and helps your body process food more efficiently. When your body is working more efficiently, you experience higher levels of energy throughout the day. You accelerate your metabolism and boost your immune system.

Weight training builds, tones, and firms up muscle. It can make women look even more feminine by creating muscular definition in just the right places and accentuating natural curves. If you are elderly, you do not have to lift a great amount of weight to derive all the benefits; you can use small amounts of weight to build your muscles back up to where they used to be. I have trained many people who are of retirement age or older. They have told me repeatedly that weight training has actually offset the aging process. They feel confident in their movement; they have regained a sense of strength, flexibility, and balance that they thought was gone forever. And I have seen hundreds of people who were extremely overweight have unbelievable success with weight training.

The Logic of Sculpting

As I mentioned at the beginning of this book, I studied infrared images while in college. I was astounded to discover that what you may know as traditional weight-training exercises largely failed to isolate a particular muscle group and work it to its full potential. Traditional weight-training exercises only work 20 to 30 percent of the targeted muscles—the top third of the muscle nearest the skin. My challenge was to reach the 70 percent of muscle that was not affected. I determined that there had to be a better way to train the body.

I began to look at the muscular structure for possible answers. I soon learned that our muscle tissue is an ever-changing entity. Seen in the light of physical transformation, muscle tissue, or lean muscle mass, is a most beneficial asset. It offsets the amount of fat we have on our bodies, boosts our metabolism, and even at rest will burn calories at a high rate. This muscle tissue is capable of almost infinite growth. Muscle tissue is made up of fibers. When you work a muscle, its fibers tear on a microscopic level. If you have ever performed a series of exercises you were not used to, it is precisely this tearing that makes you feel soreness the next day. The tearing heals, creating muscle fibers that are denser than before. This density does not necessarily mean that the muscle gets larger. When you create muscular density, more fibers exist within the same space. Muscular density occurs exponentially for a very long time before the size of the muscle actually increases. Knowing this, I felt that if I could develop a system to work the muscle from its deepest point all the way to the surface, the results would be astounding.

Using all the anatomical information available to me, I focused on the way in which the muscle is attached to the body and how the muscle enables movement. I compared these observations with our popular notions of exercise. After determining that traditional exercises were clearly invented to work particular parts of the body, I began to test their effectiveness. I quickly came to the conclusion that exercises that relied on resistance or on moving weight had the greatest potential to tap into the 70 percent of unused physical potential of most exercisers. I found that by altering existing exercises or creating entirely new exercises, I was able to develop a system that works the entire muscle. I could feel the difference when I did these exercises, but I wanted to test these theories scientifically. Again using advanced infrared technology, I studied the body with these new exercises. The images showed me that the entire muscle at work was hot!

Basic Exercise Vocabulary

As you read on, you may see a few unfamiliar words. A specific number of repetitions and a specific number of sets are prescribed in the exercises. A *repetition* is the completion of pushing or moving a weight or body part from point A to point Z. You will be instructed to perform that particular exercise for a specific number of repetitions. When you have done this, you will have completed a *set*. To maximize your effort and to truly work 100 percent of the muscle's capability, you'll need to be diligent and you'll need to concentrate.

Each exercise in the Hollywood sculpt system is designed to isolate a specific muscle or muscle group. Technically, the muscle that you target is called the *primary muscle*. Sometimes, another muscle aids the primary muscle in a movement. This helper is called the *secondary muscle*. As you'd expect, the secondary muscle does not work at 100 percent of its capability for a particular exercise. Some parts of the body are not autonomous; moving them means that several muscles or even muscle groups are involved in the motion. For example, when you throw a ball, more than just your shoulder or arm is involved in the process. You also use your legs, the muscles in your back, your chest, your abdominal muscles, and so on. These are called *tertiary muscles*. These muscles work at an even smaller percentage of their potential than the secondary muscles.

Momentumless Training

Because it is our goal to isolate the targeted muscle as much as possible, it is essential that you eliminate any extraneous movement. I call this *momentumless training*. By eliminating any swinging, throwing, or jerking movements while exercising with weights, you ensure the primary muscle is the sole focus of your work. When you swing, throw, or jerk the weight, many other muscles help you to perform the exercise. In a sense, you are cheating because you are calling upon the strength of these other muscles. You will not maximize the targeted muscle. Also, you may be cheating yourself out of the next few weeks of progress, as 90 percent of injuries occur when you swing or jerk the weights. As a trainer, one of my favorite sayings is "Bring it, don't swing it." In other words, use the targeted muscle or muscles to move the weight. But this is still only half of the exercise.

When most people work out with weights, they only concern themselves with moving the weight from a starting point to the top of that motion, or from point A to point B. But the manner in which you release the weight back to point A is the other half of the exercise that needs to be exploited to use 100 percent of the muscle's capability. When you reach point B, you will control the descent of the weight rather than letting the weight use its momentum to fall back to its point of origin. This is called the *negative*. This negative gravitational force works the muscle in the exact opposite direction. By consciously eliminating unnecessary secondary and tertiary muscle involvement and using the negative portion of the exercise, you will help yourself a great deal in achieving 100 percent of your potential.

It is impossible for a muscle to perform at 100 percent on the first repetition. For the first several repetitions of an exercise, you will not, nor would you want to, work the muscle to 100 percent of its capability. Instead, you will work your way to a muscular crescendo, a climax of performance, which happens during the last three or four repetitions of the set. These last few repetitions will and should be difficult. You should have a burning sensation as if your muscles do not have enough blood, and it should be taxing to complete these final repetitions. This is especially true of your last set in a series of exercises working any particular muscle group.

When you are performing the first two-thirds of a set of weight-training exercises, you are exercising at an aerobic level. When you enter into and complete the last third of the set, you should be reaching for and attaining an anaerobic level of exercise. You can only sustain performance at an anaerobic level for a very brief period before you have to slow down or stop. In the final repetitions of your set, you must strive to hit the anaerobic level. You will experience a shaking sensation in the muscles being worked, and you will barely be able to complete the set. The shaking of limbs, the burning sensation, the feeling that you will not be able to complete the set is really the point of the exercise.

If you could see your muscles with infrared technology at this anaerobic stage, you could clearly see the entirety of those muscles, and they would appear to be burning hot. This is the point at which you are achieving 100 percent of your muscle's capability. It makes no difference how much weight you are moving. What you are attempting to do is work the muscle into exhaustion, to a point where it is not physically able to do another repetition. In a sense, the first repetitions are a preparation for the last repetitions of the set, and the first two sets are a preparation for the last several repetitions of the last set. This is where and when results occur.

There are a few fundamental principles to achieving your goals, and it is important to understand them before your begin.

Breathing

The most fundamental action in life is breathing. Breathing is an involuntary reflex, and it is not something most people think about. It is, however, vital in weight training. Correct breathing can be a great aid in pushing through those last reps during the last set. To enlist breathing as your ally, exhale as you drive the weight; hold the weight at the top of the movement; and inhale during the negative motion on a count of three . . . two . . . one. Exhale again to move the weight, and perform the exercise in this way for the prescribed number of repetitions. This breathing method will help you move the weight. If you were to inhale as you moved the weight, your breath would actually work against you, and you might not be able to do those last repetitions.

Varying Your Routine

Most exercisers make the mistake of getting into a routine. Besides being tremendously boring, it is often the routine itself that prevents noticeable progress. The body is well equipped for adversity and even disaster. The body is designed for your survival. It will conserve as much energy as it can whenever it can. When you perform your exercises in the same way every time you work out, your body gets used to that level of exercise and will only expend the minimal amount of energy needed to perform the task.

To avoid hitting a plateau and to ensure that your body expends the greatest amount of energy possible, you must vary your workouts. Essentially, you want to outsmart your body. By changing which parts of the body you work on any given day, varying the amount of weight, and shuffling the order of exercises for each workout, you will keep your body in a state of readiness. You can constantly surprise it into performing at the highest levels possible. By varying your workout routine, you will avoid many of the pitfalls associated with training plateaus and experience the greatest results possible.

Balancing

Strive to balance your body. Work to make the left arm the same size as the right arm, the left leg the same size as the right leg, and the upper half of your body proportional to the lower half. When you work your arms and legs, focus on the weaker side. If you can do eight repetitions with the left side but fifteen with the right side, just do eight with both. Soon the left side will be as strong (and also the same size) as the right side, and you will be able to perform fifteen repetitions on each side.

Stretching

For every action, there is a reaction. When you train with weights, you use the exercise to contract a specific muscle or muscle group. After the muscle has performed at such an optimum level, you need to balance the effort by stretching the muscle out. Many people stretch before they warm up their bodies, thinking it helps prevent injury. Picture your muscles as if they were taffy. If you stretch taffy when it is cold, it will not move. If the taffy is warm, it can be stretched. Your muscles are very similar. You should only stretch *after* you have warmed them up. Because the Hollywood body system will superheat your muscles, you will have a built-in opportunity to stretch when they are the most pliable.

Some people simply rest between sets when they train with weights, but this isn't beneficial. Rather than resting, maximize your time by stretching the muscle you just worked. You will increase the blood flow to the area that just worked so hard, and the stretch will be a small reward for the muscle. Increased circulation brings needed ingredients such as oxygen, glucose, and other nutrients that nourish the muscle. Stretching the muscle after working it will offset much of the soreness you feel the next day, help to flush lactic acid out of the muscle tissue, prevent injury, and help fully develop the musculature. Aside from rewarding your body, this stretching will also affect your appearance. It will help to create beautifully elongated muscles rather than small constricted ones. For each exercise, you will find a corresponding stretch.

Resistance training with active stretching between sets becomes an aerobic activity. By not resting, the heart rate remains elevated, the metabolic rate continues to accelerate, and your muscles remain active and warm. By utilizing stretching techniques after each set of resistance training, your workout is taken to another level. Resting between sets allows the heart to slow down. Aside from wasting time, resting does little else. In contrast, when you stretch between sets, the body does not slow down significantly and the muscles continue to work.

Weight Training Tips

The single most important aspect to weight training is technique. No matter what your goals, you will not be able to attain them without a proper and nearly perfect technique. The goal is to utilize 100 percent of the muscle's capability, exhaust the muscle or muscle group, stretch it, then leave it alone. Achieving this level of performance will require you to follow the directions and photographs in this book.

Each individual has different goals that boil down to two basic strategies: (1) firming up musculature to create tone and definition and (2) adding considerable size to the muscles. You may want a combination of the two. You may want to add size to your legs and merely create some muscle tone in your chest. You may want to have bigger biceps, create size in your lateral muscles to accentuate your waist, and bring definition to your leg muscles. Although the possibilities and combinations are endless, weight training boils down to toning and shaping. The strategies for toning and shaping are similar. There are only three variables: (1) the amount of weight you are moving; (2) the number of repetitions you are moving that weight; (3) and the number of sets for each exercise.

The basic strategy for toning muscle is to perform a greater number of repetitions in the set and to work with a light or medium amount of weight. By using a relatively light weight, a greater number of repetitions will be needed to get the burn and exhaust the muscle. The strategy for creating a larger muscle is to lift a relatively heavy amount of weight. Determining the amount of weight you can or should be moving will take some experimentation. If I were standing by your side as your personal trainer, it would be quite easy for me to gauge what amount of weight you should be working with just by looking at you. Unfortunately, since I cannot be at your side, you will have to determine weight levels on your own.

Don't forget to refer to this book when you are weight lifting. If I were at your side as your personal trainer, I would demonstrate the proper technique for each exercise before you attempted it. I often demonstrate these exercises for many months, although my clients have performed them numerous times. Even if you have been exercising with weights for years, I strongly recommend that you follow the directions in this book to improve your technique each time you work out. Simply follow these directions using a weight that you feel comfortable with. Use your everyday life as a guidepost for this experimentation. (If you can pick up a gallon of milk, you know that you can safely lift 10 pounds.) Choose the lightest possible weight for the first repetition, just to get the fundamental technique of the exercise. After you are certain of the proper technique, increase the weight incrementally until you feel challenged by performing a set of ten repetitions. Perform ten repetitions of each exercise, and make a notation of the weight. This will be your starting point. From here, your transformation begins.

To attain a Hollywood body, you will reduce your body fat percentage while creating muscle definition and muscle separation. The secret to achieving these goals in the fastest possible time is learning the order with which you should work each body part, then performing the correct exercises to get the desired look.

It is said that looks are only skin deep. I disagree. It is precisely what is going on underneath the skin that can be so beautiful. Very few people exercise to get healthier. Most of us exercise to look fantastic. So let's not try to fool each other. What you are striving to accomplish is a complete physical transformation. By even attempting to embark on this journey, overwhelming changes will begin to take hold. You will bolster your confidence, raise your energy level, elevate your self-esteem, heighten your sense of accomplishment, and alter forever the manner in which you approach your life and the people you encounter. You will find no greater ally than the Hollywood sculpt system.

Your Hollywood Body Initiation— the First Two Weeks

It's time to begin the process of changing your body. What you are about to do may be difficult. I am going to push you to make several changes in your lifestyle, which might cause a slight shock to your system, but the trick to getting through this is to focus on the length of time—after all, this is only two weeks. So I'll make you a deal—a promise even; I truly believe in bottom-line results. If you do everything I suggest for two weeks and do not experience results, I'll let you off the hook and you don't have to continue. I want you to make yourself a promise, however: do everything I suggest for these first two weeks; really push yourself to get it all in every day. If you do, I promise that you will feel and see results. I promise that if you can continue to get results, you will change your life.

During these first two weeks, you will establish some new habits that will become the foundation for your transformation. By implementing Hollywood nutrition, you will break unhealthy eating cycles, eliminate food addictions, and reset your metabolism. With Hollywood heart, you will begin burning stored fat to fuel your activity. No matter what your level of physical fitness today, in two short weeks you will be ready to take on some serious challenges.

With Hollywood sculpt, you will feel the difference after your first workout; in a week, you will see the difference in the mirror; and by the end of these first two weeks, everyone will begin noticing the changes.

The Hollywood Nutrition Initiation

Your success depends on planning, which begins with your scheduling aid. As you may recall, I asked you to schedule your shopping day, I provided you with a list of foods to choose from, and I asked you to cook the protein portions in anticipation of this day. If you have done these essential tasks, congratulations—you are ready for the next step. If not, get to the store, get cooking, and get ready.

It is now time to begin scheduling your transformation. Simply open your calendar to tomorrow's date. Write down your "wake" and "sleep" times on your calendar.

You should plan to eat your first (and most important) meal of the day within an hour of rising. (If you exercise first thing in the morning, have a few bites beforehand, but understand that this is not breakfast.) Figure out the time for your first meal, and schedule "breakfast" in your calendar. You will want to eat a small snack-size meal every $2\frac{1}{2}$ to 3 hours, and you will eat at least five times, with the last meal about 2 hours before bedtime. Enter these meal times into tomorrow's ledger.

Now look over the next two weeks. The key to outthinking your starvation protection device is to be consistent with your eating schedule, reassuring this sensitive system that it does not have to store nutrients away. If you can eat at roughly the same times each day, your body will naturally relax the fat storage mechanisms and begin to release stored fat because it is no longer necessary for your survival. Using the template of your first day, eat at approximately the same times, and pencil in these eating times over the next two weeks.

Since the mid-1970s, almost every significant nutritional

advancement has been firmly rooted in the Hollywood culture. More specifically, there has not been one blockbuster diet book or phenomenal diet trend without support from at least one high-profile celebrity. All of us scour the magazine covers in the grocery store checkout line looking for the secrets of slim stars. Without this or that famous person subscribing to a particular plan, a trend, fad, or phenomenon cannot and will not occur.

Perhaps more than any other recent nutritional advancement, people have had success using high-protein/low-carb diets. Low-carb or no-carb products are available in virtually every restaurant, grocery store, and convenience store. This philosophy has changed the culture, challenged previously held beliefs on how to lose weight, and changed the food industry. Many well-known celebrities subscribe to this or similarly designed high-protein programs, and for the first two weeks I will suggest something similar.

During this two-week initiation (and only for this time period), I suggest not eating simple carbohydrates such as bread, pasta, rice, fruits, and any food product with added sugars or sweeteners (Aspartame, Saccharin, Splenda, Stevia, NutraSweet, and Equal are exceptions). Your meals will consist of protein, a selection of vegetables, and some fat.

The science behind the success of high-protein/low-carb diets suggests that when carbohydrates are eliminated from the diet, a hormonal response occurs. This response is centered on the hormone called insulin, and the elimination of these foods prevents excess insulin from being secreted into the bloodstream. The less insulin is secreted, the less fat is stored. Eating proteins will not cause insulin to be secreted; nor will the ingestion of fats. Eating carbohydrates will cause insulin secretion. After about forty-eight hours on a low-carb diet, the level of glucose (sugar) in your bloodstream will be fairly low, and you will enter a state of ketosis. This is actually the goal, for when you enter this state, your body will begin to tap into, process, and thereby eliminate fat.

Whereas many prescribe the generous intake of fats and fatty foods, I suggest the contrary. My intuition and dozens of scientific studies state that a diet of bacon and crème fraiche is not the healthiest possible thing for your heart. I actually suggest a low intake of fat. Unless you are a vegetarian, forgo dairy products such as milk, cream, yogurt, and cheese (with the exception of low-fat or no-fat cottage, string, or mozzarella cheese) during this initiation. I recommend butter substitutes, mayonnaise substitutes, nondairy alternatives without sugar, cooking sprays, and minimal use of "good" fats such as olive oil. Even these substitutes and healthy oils should be used in the most sparing manner—measured not by the teaspoon but by the drop. I suggest baking, grilling, roasting, steaming, and boiling foods, and discourage frying in oils, sautéing, and deep-frying.

During your initiation into a new way of eating, the most important step is to regain control. You are creating a new baseline for your metabolism. You are breaking the patterns that have prevented you from losing weight. You are going to retrain your taste buds and your sense of fullness, reset your internal eating clock to achieve the fat loss that must occur for you to attain a Hollywood body.

Timing

You are going to take control over your eating, and you must become very focused to overcome the patterns of behavior that have made you fatter than you want to be. In taking control, the timing of your meals is very important. If you wait too long to eat, your starvation protection device will go on alert, making fat elimination difficult if not impossible. If you can eat at roughly the same times every day, however, your body will come to trust that it will be fed regularly. It will sense that it does not have to hoard stored fat, the starvation protection device will be coaxed into a relaxed state, and your body will feel confident that it does not need all of the fat within its storage system. As a result, it will quite naturally begin to release the stored fat.

Food Selection

What and how much you eat are the other elements in retraining your body to become leaner. It is no mystery that you would gain fat if you ate only ice cream. If you flipped through any calorie counting book, you would see that fats and oils have many more calories per gram or per ounce than meats, fish, and other proteins. You know that the nutritional content of fruits and vegetables is much healthier than candies, cakes, and cookies. In fact, if you really give it some thought, you know the foods that make you fat.

How do you break the habit of eating these foods? Fast food and junk food are everywhere. Most of us crave these foods—we are addicted. Take a look at the ingredients in your favorite fast food or junk food. Chances are that you will see some ingredients you cannot pronounce. These ingredients are not natural products; they are man-made chemical compounds. While they may enhance the flavor or shelf life of foods, they may also cause cravings and addictions to them. In all cases, fast food and junk food (and the man-made chemical compounds in them) do not have enough nutritional value to sustain us. We eat more and more of them in an attempt to fulfill our hunger for nutrients. We live in a supersized society. The "extra value" of these larger sizes does nothing more than make *you* a larger size. To break this unhealthy cycle, and create the lean body you desire, you must begin eating in a precise and conscious manner.

Limit or Avoid Stimulants

Most of us start our day with caffeinated products. While caffeine may get us going, it also suppresses our appetite, dehydrates us, causes chemical imbalances, enhances sugar cravings throughout the day, and is directly related to the times of the day when our energy level seems to hit bottom. Most of us experience this energy low in the afternoon. To remain alert and energized on the job, we eat junk food. This energy low/sugar-craving cycle may happen several times during the day, and it all starts with caffeine.

If you drink coffee or strong caffeinated teas in the morning, try beginning your day with green tea. It is a potent antioxidant with many benefits. Because green tea has trace amounts of caffeine, you will not get the headaches associated with caffeine withdrawal. Switching over will also eliminate about 50 percent of food addictions and sugar cravings. To some, the taste of green tea is a little too grassy. If this is the case, simply add in some mint tea. I prefer a 3-to-1 ratio of green to mint tea, and I make it in quantity. I even put it in the refrigerator and drink it cold over ice. Do not sweeten this drink with sugar or honey, but if you must, use Splenda, Equal, or some other sugar substitute.

Your New Eating Program

To eliminate cravings, to break the cycle of food addictions, and to create a new baseline for your metabolism, you will begin eating in a new way. It will only be for two weeks. Then you will have retrained your body and established a new pattern of eating that will assist you in achieving any goal you set for yourself.

You may have nutrient and vitamin deficiencies due to former eating habits and food choices, and it is essential to correct these imbalances. You should take a daily multivitamin.

As part of each of your meals, you will have 3 to 6 ounces of protein. The protein you choose should not be processed, breaded, deep-fried, or slathered in sauces that might contain preservatives and sugars. You should use as little oil as you can when cooking these protein choices, and choose proteins that are lean such as roasted turkey, skinless chicken breasts, fish, and seafood (roasted, baked, grilled, or boiled). Try to avoid beef, dairy products, nuts (or nut products such as peanut butter), and pan-fried items that rely on too much butter or oil.

After choosing your protein for each meal, select at least an equal amount of vegetables. Again, these vegetables should be prepared with minimal oil. They are best raw, lightly steamed, or baked to a level where they retain a little crunch. The more vegetables are cooked, the more their nutrients are leeched away—unless they are in a soup, in which case the broth will be more nutritious than the vegetables themselves. The fresher the better. The closer to their natural state the better. Avoid starchy vegetables such as potatoes (red, white, gold, purple, blue), sweet potatoes, and winter squashes (acorn, butternut, spaghetti, pumpkin), and for this two-week period avoid vegetables that have a high fat content (avocado) as well as those with a high sugar content (carrots).

In addition to your protein and vegetable choices, you may have fruit. But limit your intake to 1 cup per day with the exception of berries. You may have 2 cups of berries spaced throughout the day, having them as a dessert with each meal. One cup of fruit is equal to one medium-size apple, peach, plum, or orange; half of a grapefruit; one-eighth of a cantaloupe or honeydew; two half-inch rings of pineapple; a small sliced tomato; or a portion of any other fruit that is approximately the size of your fist.

There are free foods that you may have anytime in any quantity. These foods are greens and salads using lemon or vinegar (or even salsa) as a dressing. You may have crunchy raw vegetables such as celery, cauliflower, jicama, and radishes. You may use unlimited amounts of lemon on your foods or in your drinks. Free foods also include stock vegetables (garlic, onion, bell pepper, celery), spices, and flavorings, provided that they are not overly processed and do not contain additives and preservatives. Go easy on the salt content.

One of your meals should consist of yogurt (3 ounces) or cheese and a small portion of fruit (half of an apple or half an orange, or four or five berries). One meal should be a protein drink made without sugar. For convenience I prefer to eat these meals during midmorning and midafternoon—they fit easily into a workplace setting and pace. All of your meals should contain 3 to 6 ounces of protein and some vegetables.

When the initiation has been completed, you will have reset your metabolism to the highest level, broken unhealthy cycles and eliminated cravings, and dropped up to 10 pounds of fat.

Helpful Nutrition Tips

▌ Drink a lot of water. All guidelines suggest drinking at least eight glasses (64 ounces) of water each day. Not only will this keep you hydrated, but it will also help you feel more full, flush toxins and lactic acid, and speed the elimination of body fat.

▌ Reduce your caffeine intake. The nutritional objective in these first two weeks is to lead your body into a state of ketosis. Caffeine (especially in the form of coffee) may impede this process. If you are a coffee drinker, start your day with green tea. The longer your tea is steeped in hot water the more concentrated it becomes. Drinking green tea or the green tea–mint tea combination that I recommend in the morning will enable you to escape the headaches and sluggishness associated with caffeine withdrawal. If you must have coffee, have a cup of decaffeinated coffee as part of your midmorning break. You could also have a noncaffeinated hot or iced tea between or right after your meals. Tea is available in many flavors, so if you have a sweet tooth, get yourself a variety of flavored teas to substitute for sweet treats. If you have a glass of water or a cup of hot tea after your meals, you will feel more satisfied and full.

▌ Be prepared for the effects of low blood sugar. Eating every $2^{1}/_{2}$ to 3 hours during this initiation phase is essential. It has been reported that some people get edgy, crabby, and even a little weak or nauseated when their blood sugar falls below a certain level. Since you will not be eating a great deal of food at one sitting and that food will not contain the amount of carbohydrates you may be used to, it may be necessary to eat more frequently than I have previously suggested. Always keep a protein drink, an apple, some veggies, some raw nuts, or low-fat packaged cheese with you. If you feel your meals need to be closer together, make the adjustments you require.

■ When eating out, do yourself the favor of immediately asking your server to bring you a salad or a bowl of vegetable soup instead of a basket of bread. Instead of the usual serving of starch (potatoes, pasta, or rice), ask for a double serving of vegetables. Remember that the sauces that come on meats, fish, vegetables, and salads contain sugar, additives, and preservatives. These products will take you out of ketosis. Ask for sauces on the side, and use them very sparingly if at all. The less processed foods you eat the better. The cleaner the cooking method (the lower the fat content) the better.

The Hollywood Heart Initiation

It is estimated that less than 10 percent of the population exercises regularly. These next two weeks are going to be a very exciting time. You are about to discover that cardiovascular activity can do much more than shrink your waist.

If you haven't exercised for some time, your endurance will improve exponentially each day. You are going to elevate your fitness level in a short amount of time. In just two short weeks, the objective is to be fit enough to take on the physical challenges needed to make dramatic changes to your appearance. An even greater goal is to embark upon a fitness regimen that will maximize your heart health. Like the biceps, calves, and thighs, your heart is a muscle that can be conditioned and strengthened. Unlike the biceps, calves, and thighs, the muscles that allow your heart to function as an organ are essential for your survival. Wherever you are today, you can improve your heart health to the highest possible level within six months.

Assuming you have never exercised or have not exercised for some time, the idea is to keep this as simple and as pain-free as you can. The primary goal is to raise your level of fitness and increase your stamina and endurance. You need to begin slowly and work your way up. I have had several clients who had never exercised before and are now running marathons. When they first started exercising, the goal of completing a 26-mile race seemed impossible. All of them began by walking. Slowly, they inserted a one-block jog into their walk. They worked their way up to two, then three blocks of jogging during their walking session. Soon those blocks turned into miles. While you may or may not be up to conditioning yourself in a similar manner, the point is that you need to begin gradually as you challenge yourself to go for longer distances with more and more intensity.

On days that you work with weights, perform your cardiovascular session after your strength-training session. I have found that this is a fantastic prescription for offsetting muscular soreness (especially in your legs) and providing a sense of completion. Keep in mind that the complete workout (strength and cardio) should take less than an hour to perform. If you don't have a full hour, you may split it up and spend approximately 20 minutes on your Hollywood sculpt program and at least 25 minutes walking in two separate time blocks.

With these approximate time considerations in mind, open your calendar to tomorrow's date. Pencil in a 30-minute appointment for your cardio session. Some people prefer to do their cardiovascular exercise after work or dinner, or after they put the kids to sleep. Some exercisers make this one small time segment their own sanctuary of peace and serenity. The people who choose to exercise in the evening generally find that it clears their heads, allows them to focus, and relaxes them sufficiently to begin to wind down their day. Some people prefer this exercise in the morning to give them an energy boost that sets the tone for a positive day. If you have trouble finding time, the morning session may be for you, even if you have to set your alarm clock a little earlier.

After you have completed this initiation phase of cardiovascular exercise, I hope it will become the most essential and valuable portion of your day. In anticipation of giving yourself the greatest gift of your life, schedule in five additional days that you will exercise in your first week of initiation. Now schedule in one day that you will rest and let your body rejuvenate. Block off that entire day. While I would not discourage you from shooting a round of golf or working in the yard on your rest day, it should be a day off from strength and cardio work.

Now look at week two. Schedule in six days that you will do at least 25 consecutive minutes of cardiovascular exercise. If something comes up, move this session around (that's why it is in pencil), but do not get in bed without honoring your commitment to yourself. Schedule in a day of rest and rejuvenation.

Here are some important items to get before beginning the cardiovascular program:

- A heart rate monitor (optional)
- A good pair of cross-training athletic shoes
- Comfortable clothing that you can move in
- A spiral-bound weekly schedule, day planner, or electronic scheduling aid
- A good-quality multivitamin
- A 32-ounce water bottle

Cardiovascular Timing

You only need to spend 25 minutes on your cardio workout. According to the Centers for Disease Control, to improve your heart health and strengthen the muscles that comprise the organ of your heart, you need at least 25 minutes of exercise. By following the Hollywood nutrition principles, you will have a relatively small amount of nutrients in your bloodstream at any given time. Once those nutrients have been depleted, your body must tap into its reserve tank (fat) to fuel your activity. You will use up all the nutrients in your bloodstream within the first 10 to 15 minutes, so for the duration of your session the rest of the calories (energy) you burn will come from stored fat. (This burn rate is most efficient when you elevate your heart rate to the 70 percent level, and these first two weeks are the preparation to be able to achieve this level of exercise.) The energy and nutrients stored within your fat cells can only be tapped for so long before your body refuses to give up more. Therefore, after about an hour (really an hour and fifteen minutes) you will have maximized the amount of fat that can be expended in this session. So walk for at least 25 consecutive minutes, and keep your walk under an hour and a half.

Walking Guidelines

For the first two weeks, your program is fairly simple. Six days a week, you are going to take a walk. This walk will last at least 25 consecutive minutes. If you have to cross a street and wait for traffic, walk in place and swing your arms. Keep your heart rate elevated sufficiently. Remember that your heart rate monitor is a very helpful tool that will confirm you are walking at a rate that is burning the most amount of fat in the least amount of time. Keep your heart rate between 60 percent and 70 percent of your maximum.

Do not take the same walking route on two consecutive days. The objective is to surprise your body on a daily basis. If you do the same thing day after day, your body will quickly adapt and conserve all the energy it can, and you will fail to see results. Try to have four or five different routes. Walk through locations where the terrain varies and you are forced to encounter hills or places where the grade gets steeper. Not only will this work a wider variety of muscle groups, but the pace and intensity of your walk will be varied. If you do your cardiovascular workouts on a treadmill, vary the incline level, which will force you to increase and decrease your pace. If you use machinery, never follow the same program for two consecutive days.

To work your way up to your 70 percent heart rate level, it may be helpful to jot down these daily objectives in the time block you have already scheduled in your calendar:

Days 1 through 4: 25 minutes at 60 percent of your maximum heart rate

Days 5 through 7: 25 minutes between 60 and 65 percent of your maximum heart rate

Days 8 and 9: 25 minutes at 70 percent of your maximum heart rate

Days 10 through 12: 25 minutes at 75 percent of your maximum heart rate

Helpful Cardiovascular Tips

▌ Push yourself a little more every day. During these first two weeks, do not increase the duration of your session by more than five minutes from the previous day. Do not walk more than six blocks farther than you did the previous day. And do not increase your heart rate level by more than 5 percent over the previous day's session. It is better to gradually increase than to overexert yourself, burn out, and quit.

▌ Do not take the same route on two consecutive days. Establish several routes, then discover more with varying terrain. If you feel up for a challenge, use the route with more hills. Surprise your body every day, and you will have the greatest results.

▌ If you are walking alone, consider investing in a portable music player or radio with headphones. Listening to music or the news makes the time go by faster. Instead of reading the morning paper, I get my news by radio during my morning cardio session.

▌ You will soon discover that the time you spend exercising your heart and burning fat is true quality time, and you just might want to share that time with someone special. Bring along a loved one, a friend, a neighbor, or a colleague from work. This may be the most creative portion of your day. The person you share this time with might be the catalyst for your latest breakthrough or your next blockbuster idea.

▌ Take one day off each week to rest and allow your body to rejuvenate.

The Hollywood Sculpt Initiation

As I have said, the Hollywood body is really the sum of many parts. I will not reiterate the goals and target body areas. But remember that the basic overview of my revolutionary system is that you will reshape each and every muscle from its deepest point so that you will look (and be) dramatically different when you complete the program. The Hollywood body represents a road map for a total body makeover.

You will create muscular density, not muscular mass, size, or bulk. Muscle weighs approximately two times more than fat. When you create more muscle, you automatically reduce your body fat percentage. So let's say that you lose 5 to 10 pounds of body fat over the next two weeks by combining the Hollywood nutrition and Hollywood heart principles, and you gain 1 or 2 pounds of muscle over the same period using Hollywood sculpt. The scale will tell you that you are 3 to 8 pounds lighter, but in fact you may have lowered your body fat by as much as 10 percent. Your body fat measurement will tell you your total weight, define how much or what percentage of that weight is made up of lean muscle, bone, hair, and so on, and how many pounds of your total weight is fat. The goal is to continually reduce the portion of your weight that is fat and increase the percentage that is made up of the good stuff.

When you increase the percentage of lean muscle mass, you are doing much more than improving your appearance. You are improving your metabolism, immune function, and overall health as well as your skeletal strength, structure, and functionality. Do you know people who can eat anything they want without gaining weight? Their secret is lean muscle mass. Muscle consumes more energy (calories) than fat. As you increase the percentage of lean muscle mass, you will burn more calories, even when you are at rest. This increase in lean muscle will positively enhance your metabolism, and your body will essentially become a calorie-burning furnace.

Lean muscle mass will create a better support structure for your skeletal system. More of my new clients come in with significant structural problems. Because of the changing dynamics in technology and in the workplace, most of us spend long hours hunched over a keyboard looking at a computer monitor. Just as redundancy can cause injuries and ailments for factory workers who spend the majority of the day doing one specific task, long periods of sitting at a desk and typing will cause posture-related ailments, which can gradually affect skeletal structure. Much of my initial work with new clients is focused on correcting the muscular weakness and atrophy that contributes to poor posture, imbalance, and other bone-related issues that can cause a great deal of pain and discomfort. As you embark on these first two weeks of initiation, the goal is to move toward correcting structural challenges.

Strength Planning

Reshaping every muscle in your body in order to experience a complete body makeover will require time and effort. During this two-week initiation, you will perform my Hollywood sculpt routines three times per week.

Open your calendar to tomorrow's date. Schedule in three 25-minute blocks over the first week, ideally every other day. If possible, each of these sessions should be followed immediately by your cardiovascular session. Once you have scheduled your first week of sessions, schedule in three sessions for your second week.

These appointments to exercise represent a commitment and a promise you have made to yourself. Try to give these appointments the same priority as other important events in your life.

The Timing of Toning

While it does not matter what time of the day you exercise, your timing matters a great deal during these revolutionary exercises. If you have worked out before, you will notice that these exercises are designed to be performed more slowly than traditional ones. The objective is to isolate the targeted muscle or muscle group as much as possible and work it to exhaustion (a point where you can no longer move the weight).

There is a particular cadence involved with each exercise. First, you exhale and move the weight with an explosive movement on a count of one. Then you hold the weight as you finish your exhalation. Next, you inhale, and on a count of three . . . two . . . one, you bring the weight back to the starting position in a very controlled manner. (This is called the "negative" portion of the exercise and works the targeted muscle in the opposite direction.) Finally, you hold the weight in the starting position as you finish your inhalation. Your primary focus is to perform each repetition of each exercise to perfection, maintaining perfect form and perfect technique. By using this formula for your timing, not only will you be better able to focus on the task at hand, but you will also discover some mental benefits. When you learn to breathe and move as I have directed, you will discover the Zen of toning. You will quickly find that this particular block of time takes you to another state of consciousness and positively alters your headspace.

Getting Started

I have designed each session to replicate the experience of having me by your side as your personal trainer. Remember that the objective is to perform each repetition of each exercise with perfect technique and form. To help my clients, I always demonstrate the exercise before they begin, regardless of how long we have been working together. They pick up some subtle nuances when I do this. Since I cannot be there to personally demonstrate these exercises for you, page references in the exercise tables beginning on page 90 will tell you where to find the description and photographic demonstration of each exercise.

You will notice that each exercise prescribes a specific number of repetitions in each set. After you have completed the set, there is also a stretch to be performed immediately (without stopping to rest). Not only will the stretch create beautiful, elongated musculature, but it will also keep your heart rate at a certain level so that the entire program becomes an aerobic session. When you have completed the stretch, you will immediately return to perform the next set or move on to the next exercise.

You will feel the difference in your body after your first workout. After the first week, you may see the changes when you look in the mirror. By the time you finish your second week, others will begin to notice the changes.

Helpful Training Tips

- Every personal client of mine is required to warm up before they begin strength training. In the gym setting, they are required to get on the treadmill, elliptical trainer, or stationary bike and do five minutes of cardiovascular activity. You should do something to get your circulation pumping, warm up your muscles, and get yourself prepared to work out. If you can't get outdoors to get in a quick power walk, perhaps you can skip rope, do some calisthenics, or march in place for five minutes. It is essential to do this to prevent injury and to get the results you are looking for.

- You are strategically setting yourself up for muscular failure with every exercise. When you reach the point where your arms or legs are shaking, when you feel that you just can't move the weight, when your body will not allow you to do another repetition, you have reached the result zone. This is the goal. With every repetition you are preparing for this event. The first and second sets prepare you for the third set, and in the final repetitions of the last set, the magic begins to happen. If your muscles fail, you haven't. You are a success when your muscles fail.

- Always finish the set. If you have to drop the weight, by all means switch to a lower set of weights, but finish the set.

- To isolate the targeted muscle as much as possible, use the principles of momentumless training. Do not swing the weights or jerk your body to help you move the weights. Bring it, don't swing it.

■ There is a distinct possibility that you might experience some muscular soreness, especially if it has been a while since you last exercised. Realize that there is a difference between feeling soreness and having an injury. These exercises were designed to severely limit the possibility of injury and to be the safest possible exercise options. If you ever experience a torn muscle or ligament, it is wise to discontinue exercise. But the best course of action to combat sore muscles is to work them again (even if this may seem counterintuitive). When you exercise, your body produces a substance called lactic acid. It is not truly a liquid but rather a crystalline substance with sharp and jagged edges that lodges between muscle fibers. When you move, you are feeling the effects of these sharp and jagged edges. To flush this lactic acid, drink plenty of water, and be sure to get in your daily walk. If you are still uncomfortable, you may find that a hot bath with a generous amount of Epsom salts alleviates the symptoms. Still sore? Try plopping two tablets of Alka-Seltzer Plus in a glass of water. If you prefer natural remedies, it has been reported that fresh pineapple also does the trick (just be sure to eat some low-fat cheese along with it).

TONING INITIATION FOR WOMEN

Perform two sets of 20 repetitions. Stretch after each set.

DAY 1	Page	DAY 2	Page	DAY 3	Page
Ball Squat	98	Butt Lift	103	Arrow	95
Side Kick	102	Inner Thigh	96	Leg Curl	97
Bent-Over Row	105	Squat Curl	134	Cheer	115
Wings	116	Incline Fly	120	Pull-In	109
Kickback	130	Overhead Tri	132	Ball Curl	138
Squeeze	144	Ball Crunch	141	Corkscrew	149
Penguin	147	Side Raise	150	Crunch	145
Ball Small Sit-Up	142	Crossover Crunch	146	Leg Lift	148

DAY 4	Page	DAY 5	Page	DAY 6	Page
Kickout	129	Reverse Lunge	94	Ball Lunge	101
C Sweep	123	Butt Lift	103	Arrow	95
Pull-Over	107	Calf Raise	99	Beginner Push-Up	124
Lunge	93	Bent-Over Row	105	Dip	133
Side Kick	102	Karate Curl	139	Cross-Curl	137
Ball Pike	143	Leg Lift	148	Ball Crunch	141
Lying Side Raise	151	Penguin	147	Corkscrew	149
Crossover Crunch	146	Ball Small Sit-Up	142	Squeeze	144

TONING INITIATION FOR MEN

Perform two sets of 15 repetitions. Stretch after each set.

DAY 1	Page	DAY 2	Page	DAY 3	Page
Advanced Push-Up	125	Lunge	93	Incline Fly	120
Bent-Over Row	105	Arrow	95	Kickback	130
W Shoulders	112	Tricep Extension	128	One-Arm Row	106
Tricep Extension	128	Wave	117	Overhead Tri	132
Squat Curl	134	C Sweep	123	Ball Curl	138
Leg Curl	97	Hammer Curl	136	Ball Squat	98
Crunch	145	Squeeze	144	Corkscrew	149
Penguin	147	Side Raise	150	Leg Lift	148
Ball Small Sit-Up	142	Crossover Crunch	146	Lying Side Raise	151

DAY 4	Page	DAY 5	Page	DAY 6	Page
Reverse Lunge	94	Decline Push-Up	121	Cheer	115
Calf Raise	99	Kickout	129	Kickbacks	130
Fly	119	Rear Delt	114	Ball Push-Up	126
Twisting W	113	Pull-In	109	Pull-Over	107
Dip	133	Squat Curl	134	Hammer Curl	136
Karate Curl	139	Lunge	93	Leg Curl	97
Ball Crunch	141	Ball Crunch	141	Ball Pike	143
Penguin	147	Side Raise	150	Leg Lift	148
Ball Small Sit-Up	142	Squeeze	144	Corkscrew	149

The Exercises

Hollywood Legs

Hollywood legs strive to achieve four things. First, the thigh muscles should be long and defined, tapering down as the muscles connect with the knee. Second, these quadricep muscles should be strengthened and toned so that you can see each one of them. In the highly trained state, a line appears down the center of the thigh like a crisply ironed pair of pants. Third and most important, rather than a straight line reaching from the back of the knee toward the buttocks, this line should bow slightly. Fourth, the calf muscles require development; the more toned and defined these muscles become, the more the eye is drawn to them. Aside from deemphasizing thick ankles, the development of your calf muscles will create a balance in relationship to your thighs and upper arms. To balance the size of each thigh, exercises are performed one leg at a time.

The leg muscles are the largest in your body and are of primary importance. Working this large group of muscles jump-starts a chain reaction of physical results throughout the rest of the body.

☆ Hollywood Lunge

The walking lunge is one of the finest exercises for creating shape from the waist down. You will really feel this exercise in the buttocks and thighs. It is designed to be an effective warm-up for all the muscles in the legs, and it's great for beginning or ending your leg workout. The walking lunge can be performed to accommodate any level of fitness.

GET READY

BEGINNER: With your legs 3 inches apart, stand with your hands on your hips.

ADVANCED: With your legs 3 inches apart, stand with a dumbbell in each hand. Allow your arms to be fully extended, with your hands hanging down next to your thighs. They will remain

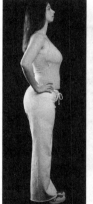 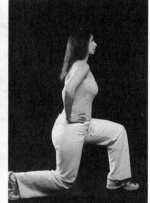

in this position throughout the exercise. The more advanced you become, the greater the weight.

THE EXERCISE

From the standing position, inhale and step forward with your left leg, landing on your heel. With your left foot flat against the ground, bend your left knee until it is at a 90 degree angle. Keep the torso straight and allow the right heel to rise as you lower your body until you can almost touch the ground with your right knee. Exhale and return to standing, pressing through the left heel. When your legs are fully extended, bring the feet together and repeat with your right leg. Perform the prescribed number of paces, alternating legs, and stretch after each set.

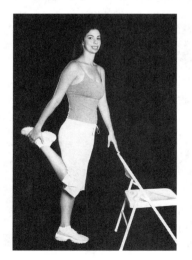

FRONT STRETCH

Standing with your feet together, lift your right heel back toward your buttocks. If you need to, you may use your left hand to balance or brace yourself against something sturdy. Holding your right ankle with your right hand, bring the heel closer toward the buttocks. Continue stretching for 30 seconds. Repeat on the left side.

Hollywood Reverse Lunge

GET READY

Stand upright, with your feet about hip-width apart.

THE EXERCISE

From the standing position, inhale, and step back with your right leg so that only the ball of the right foot is touching the floor. Bend your left knee, lowering yourself down as far as you can without touching, so that your left knee is bent at a 90-degree angle. the knee should not extend beyond the toes. Exhale and come back up into the starting position and repeat with the left leg. Repeat the prescribed number of repetitions, alternating legs, and stretch after each set using the front stretch.

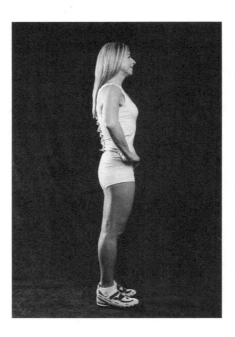
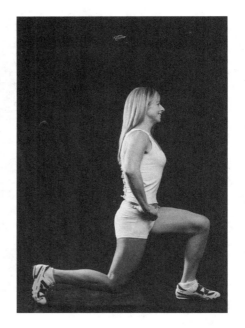

FRONT STRETCH

Standing with your feet together, lift your right heel back toward your buttocks (see photo on page 93). If you need to, you may use your left hand to balance or brace yourself against something sturdy. Holding your right ankle with your right hand, bring the heel closer toward the buttocks. Continue stretching for 30 seconds. Repeat on the left side.

⭐ Hollywood Arrow

GET READY

As you first begin doing this exercise, place a chair 2 to 3 feet in front of you. Turn the chair to the side so that you can use the back or seat for support. As you become more advanced, the goal will be to perform this exercise without any support.

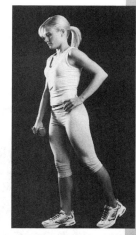

Stand up tall and lock your knees. Your feet should be separated slightly, no farther than hip-width apart. Your left hand is on the chair, your right hand holds a dumbbell. Allow your right arm to relax and hang toward the floor throughout the exercise.

THE EXERCISE

Exhale and reach backward with your left heel. Keep your left leg and torso completely straight and rigid. You are one straight line from your foot to your head. Tilt forward slowly until you are parallel to the floor and perpendicular to your right leg. Stop and hold for one count as you finish your exhalation. Inhale and slowly return to the starting position on a count of three . . . two . . .

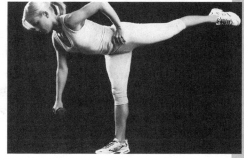

one. Switch legs and repeat. Repeat for the prescribed number of repetitions. Stretch after each set using the ragdoll stretch.

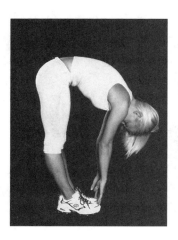

RAGDOLL STRETCH

Stand up tall with your arms at your sides. Drop your chin to your chest. Let the weight of your head pull you down vertebra by vertebra. Allow your arms to hang down so that your fingers are pointing toward your toes. Touch your toes, or come as close as your hamstrings will allow you to. If you can easily touch your toes, try to touch the palms of your hands against the floor. If you are especially limber, cross your arms and try to touch your elbows to the floor. Above all, keep the motion constant and avoid bouncing. Maintain this continuous stretch and try to deepen it for at least 30 seconds.

☆ Hollywood Inner Thigh

GET READY

Using ankle weights, lie down on your left side. Bend your right knee and place your foot firmly on the floor in front of your left knee. You should be in one straight line from your head to your left foot. Flex your left foot and lock your left knee.

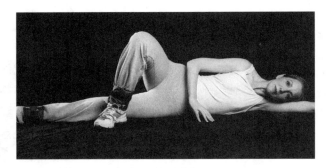

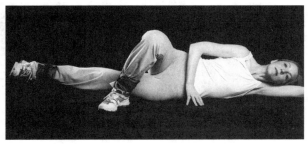

THE EXERCISE

Exhale and lift your left leg up as high as you possibly can on a one count. Hold at the top of the movement as you finish your exhalation. With your knee still locked, lower your ankle to the ground slowly on a count of two . . . one. Do the prescribed number of repetitions on each leg and stretch after each set using the butterfly stretch.

BUTTERFLY STRETCH

Come up into a sitting position, and bring the soles of your feet together. Pull your heels toward you as far as you comfortably can. Push down on your knees and hold for 20 seconds. Spread your legs as wide as you comfortably can. With your back straight, hold this stretch for 20 seconds.

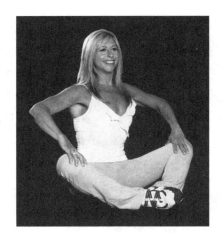

★ Hollywood Leg Curl

GET READY

With weights on each of your ankles, stand behind a chair. Place one of your hands on top of the chair back for support.

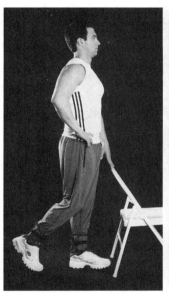 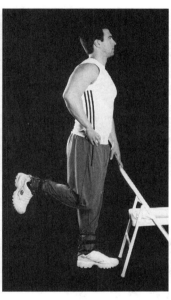

THE EXERCISE

Exhale and lift your right heel up toward your buttocks slowly on a count of three . . . two . . . one. Do not let your knee move forward as you lift. Hold at the top of the movement as you finish your exhalation while you contract the thigh muscle as much as possible. Inhale and slowly release your foot back down to the starting position on a count of three . . . two . . . one. Repeat the prescribed number of repetitions and stretch after each set using the ragdoll stretch.

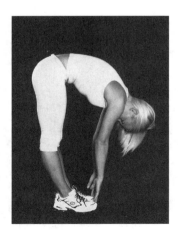

RAGDOLL STRETCH

Stand up tall with your arms at your sides. Drop your chin to your chest. Let the weight of your head pull you down vertebra by vertebra. Allow your arms to hang down so that your fingers are pointing toward your toes. Touch your toes, or come as close as your hamstrings will allow you to. If you can easily touch your toes, try to touch the palms of your hands against the floor. If you are especially limber, cross your arms and try to touch your elbows to the floor. Above all, keep the motion constant and avoid bouncing. Maintain this continuous stretch and try to deepen it for at least 30 seconds.

⭐ Hollywood Ball Squat

GET READY

Find a sturdy wall. Stand with your back to the wall and position your exercise ball behind the small of your back. Walk your feet out slightly. Your legs should be shoulder-width apart and your feet should be turned out. Plant your feet firmly on the floor.

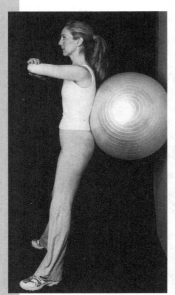 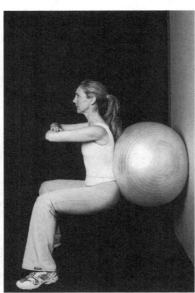

THE EXERCISE

Inhale and slowly lower your buttocks toward the floor until your legs are at a 90-degree angle, allowing the exercise ball to roll up your spine as your pelvis tilts back toward the wall. Do not allow your knees to extend over your toes. Exhale, and in an explosive movement, come back to your starting position. Repeat the prescribed number of repetitions and stretch after each set using the ragdoll stretch.

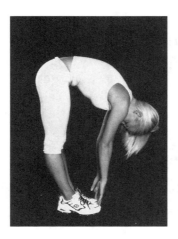

RAGDOLL STRETCH

Stand up tall with your arms at your sides. Drop your chin to your chest. Let the weight of your head pull you down vertebra by vertebra. Allow your arms to hang down so that your fingers are pointing toward your toes. Touch your toes, or come as close as your hamstrings will allow you to. If you can easily touch your toes, try to touch the palms of your hands against the floor. If you are especially limber, cross your arms and try to touch your elbows to the floor. Above all, keep the motion constant and avoid bouncing. Maintain this continuous stretch and try to deepen it for at least 30 seconds.

☆ Hollywood Calf Raise

GET READY

Find a raised object such as a stair, a step used for aerobics, a platform without a lip, or even a low bench. Stand on top of the object in such a way that your heels are unimpeded. Move back so that the only contact point between your foot and the object you are standing on are the balls of your feet and your toes. Allow the heels to lower as far as possible, and feel the stretch through the back of your calves. Hold onto something for balance, but do not support your weight with that object.

THE EXERCISE

Allow your heels to sink as far as they possibly can. Exhale and drive up until you are standing tippy-toed on the balls of your feet. Inhale and lower yourself down on a count of three . . . two . . . one as your heels reach toward the floor. Hold at the bottom for one count and feel the stretch through the back of your calves as you finish your exhalation. Exhale and repeat the movement for the prescribed number of repetitions, and stretch after each set using the calf stretch.

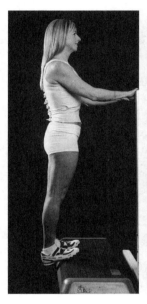 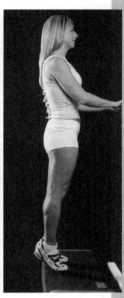

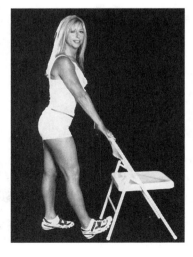

CALF STRETCH

Stand facing the back of a chair. Place your hands on top of the chair for balance, and stand up straight. Lean back slightly while you place your right heel near the rear right leg of the chair. Tilt back farther and place your right foot on the leg of the chair. Stand up straight and stretch for 15 seconds. Repeat on the left side.

Hollywood Hips

No longer do Hollywood bodies have the waiflike hips and unattainable buttocks of runway models. Today's stars have shapely, rounded buttocks that closely resemble those of an athlete. Look at the backside of Jessica Simpson, watch *Charlie's Angels: Full Throttle* (where Cameron Diaz's derriere should have had a costar credit), or check out Jennifer Lopez's caboose to see that size truly does not matter. What is of major concern is the shape, firmness, and form of your posterior.

A teardrop booty is not just for women. For men and women alike, shapely buttocks truly finish the look and line of the legs, complement the way the lower half of the body looks, and set the stage for creating a complete and balanced look with the upper half of the body. What you are looking to achieve here is the delineation between the uppermost thigh and the bottom of the buttock, and a more athletically rounded buttock with a dimple on each side.

When seen in profile, the well-developed buttock will have an almost teardrop-like shape. This more prominent look can help camouflage many other areas of concern. Some people have wide hips. Developing the shape of these muscles will not only eliminate the flatter backside but will also make wide hips appear to be better proportioned, consequently deemphasizing size-related issues.

Hollywood Ball Lunge

GET READY

With a chair in front of you and your exercise ball 2 to 3 feet behind you, stand upright and place your right foot on top of the ball. Bend your knees, lean forward, and hold onto the chair. Keep your knees soft. Position the ball on your shin between your right knee and ankle. Balance yourself so that you feel stable.

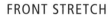

THE EXERCISE

Inhale and bend your left knee to a 90-degree angle. Do not let your bent knee extend over your toes. Hold for a brief moment. Exhale, and with an explosive movement, return to your starting position. Repeat the prescribed number of repetitions, and repeat on the other side. Stretch after each set using the front stretch.

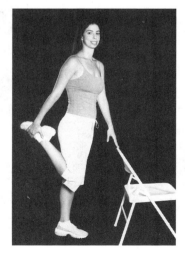

FRONT STRETCH

Standing with your feet together, lift your right heel back toward your buttocks. If you need to, you may use your left hand to balance or brace yourself against something sturdy. Holding your right ankle with your right hand, bring the heel closer toward the buttocks. Continue stretching for 30 seconds. Repeat on the left side.

⭐ Hollywood Side Kick

GET READY

You may want to use a mat, a carpeted floor, or a rug. Lie down on your left side. Extend your left arm so your head is resting against it. You should be in one straight line from your fingers to your toes. Lift your right leg up 12 to 18 inches. You may place your right hand on the floor for support.

THE EXERCISE

Inhale, bend your right knee, and bring it up toward or into your chest. Hold for a brief moment. Exhale, and pushing through your heel, extend your right leg until it is straight. Then lift it up until it is at a 45-degree angle. Repeat the prescribed number of repetitions, then repeat on the other side and stretch after each set using the hip stretch.

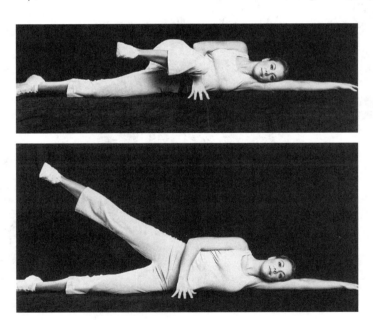

HIP STRETCH

Sit on the floor with your legs in front of you. Bend your right knee, lift it up and over the left, and place your foot just outside your left knee (see photo on page 103). Place your left hand on the outside of your right knee and pull it toward your left shoulder. Try to deepen the stretch for at least 20 seconds. Repeat on the other side.

⭐ Hollywood Butt Lift

This exercise is a fantastic tool to create separation and delineation between the hamstring muscles and the buttocks.

GET READY

Place your exercise ball against the wall. Lie on your back, and with your buttocks about a foot in front of the ball, place your left heel near the top of the ball. Cross your right leg over your left so that your right ankle is on top of or just below your left knee. Your hands are at your sides with your palms against the floor.

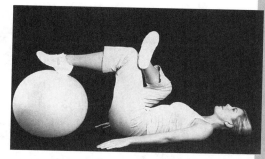

THE EXERCISE

Exhale, and pushing through your left heel, lift your buttocks 6 to 10 inches off the ground. Inhale and come back down to the starting position on a count of three . . . two . . . one. Perform the prescribed number of repetitions and repeat on the other side, stretching after each set using the hip stretch.

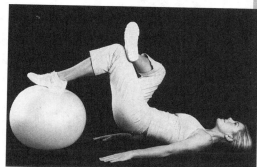

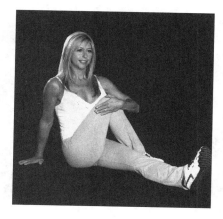

HIP STRETCH

Sit on the floor with your legs in front of you. Bend your right knee, lift it up and over the left, and place your foot just outside your left knee. Place your left hand on the outside of your right knee and pull it toward your left shoulder. Try to deepen the stretch for at least 20 seconds. Repeat on the other side.

Hollywood Back

The development of back muscles is very important. For both men and women, a well-defined back contributes to a sexy and sensuous allure.

A well-developed back is the key to appearing longer through the torso, which will enable you to camouflage many areas of the body that you are less than pleased with. To deemphasize a thick waist, wide hips, or a square physique, particular attention must be paid to the back, especially the lateral muscles, which are the winglike muscles of your back that start below your armpits and reach down to the middle of your ribs. If you can increase the tone or even the size of these muscles, you can do much to create a sensually athletic hourglass curve.

⭐ Hollywood Bent-Over Row

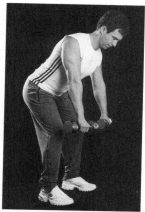

GET READY

This exercise is performed in two movements that are designed to work the shoulder blades and the middle portion of your back. Flexing the muscles in your back is the first and most important part of the exercise. This is not a workout for your arms. The point is to depend more on back muscles. To maximize the muscles in the upper back, you will engage the shoulder blades by flexing the back or squeezing the shoulder blades together.

Standing with your feet shoulder-width apart and a dumbbell in each hand, bend your knees and squat slightly, as if you were beginning to sit down in a chair. With your back straight, lean forward slightly.

THE EXERCISE

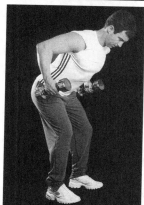

First, exhale as you engage the shoulder blades by flexing the back, or squeezing the shoulder blades together. Then, bring the dumbbells up as high as you possibly can so that your elbows are pointed toward the ceiling. Hold for a count of one. Inhale on a count of three . . . two . . . one, easing the weight back toward your starting position until your arms are fully extended. Release the flex in your back muscles and let the weight pull your torso forward until you are enjoying a nice stretch along your back. Exhale and repeat for the prescribed number of repetitions, and stretch after each set using the back stretch.

BACK STRETCH

Find a pole that is solid enough to support your weight. Facing the pole, place your feet on either side of its base. Interlock your fingers around the pole and place your hands above your head. Let the weight of your buttocks and torso fall away from the pole and allow your body to form the shape of an archer's bow. Feel the stretch between your shoulder blades and along the length of your back. Perform this stretch for 40 seconds after each set.

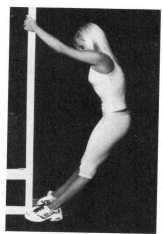

☆ Hollywood One-Arm Row

This exercise will develop your back and promote a muscular balance between your right and left sides. As in the bent-over row, particular attention should be paid to engaging the shoulder blades.

GET READY

This exercise is performed using one dumbbell. With your exercise ball approximately 2 feet in front of you, bend at the waist until your back is flat. Place your left hand on top of the ball for stability. Extend your right hand and grip the dumbbell. Feel the weight gently stretch the muscles along your right shoulder blade. Keeping your right arm straight and long, engage the right shoulder.

THE EXERCISE

Exhale, and with an explosive motion, bring the right elbow up and above your back until it is pointed straight at the ceiling. The motion is like sawing a piece of wood. Hold this position for one count. Inhale and lower the weight toward the floor on a count of three . . . two . . . one. Feel the stretch through your back and shoulder as you finish your inhalation. Repeat the prescribed number of repetitions, and repeat the same number on your left side. Remember to work to the weak side for muscular balance. Stretch after each set using the back stretch.

BACK STRETCH

Find a pole that is solid enough to support your weight. Facing the pole, place your feet on either side of its base. Interlock your fingers around the pole and place your hands above your head. Let the weight of your buttocks and torso fall away from the pole and allow your body to form the shape of an archer's bow (see photo on page 107). Feel the stretch between your shoulder blades and along the length of your back. Perform this stretch for 40 seconds after each set.

★ Hollywood Pull-Over

GET READY

With a dumbbell in each hand, lie back on your exercise ball, positioning the ball in the middle of your back underneath your shoulder blades. Press the dumbbells up toward the ceiling so that your arms are straight but the elbows are not locked.

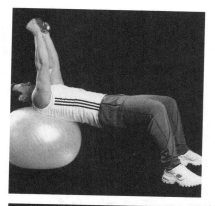

THE EXERCISE

Inhale and slowly bring the dumbbells over your head as far as you can on a count of three . . . two . . . one. Hold for a moment as you finish your inhalation. Exhale and pull your arms back up to the starting position on a count of one . . . two. Hold, and finish your exhalation. Perform the prescribed number of repetitions, and stretch after each set using the back stretch.

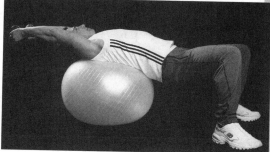

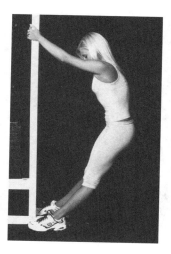

BACK STRETCH

Find a pole that is solid enough to support your weight. Facing the pole, place your feet on either side of its base. Interlock your fingers around the pole and place your hands above your head. Let the weight of your buttocks and torso fall away from the pole and allow your body to form the shape of an archer's bow. Feel the stretch between your shoulder blades and along the length of your back. Perform this stretch for 40 seconds after each set.

☆ Hollywood Hyperextension

The hyperextension is one of the most fantastic exercises for the lower back. It will improve your posture. It is a fantastic exercise for those with back problems, those with weakness in the lower back, and those who have suffered a back injury. The hyperextension could also prevent injury and improve the strength and appearance of your abdominal muscles.

The movement for this exercise is not an explosive one. Maintain a slow and even pace. The motion should be fluid and without jerking movements.

GET READY
With your exercise ball on the floor, kneel beside it and place your tummy on the ball. Bring your arms over the ball, and roll forward slowly until your body is draped over the ball. Bring your knees up off the ground, and place the soles of your feet against a wall if you need to. Stay there for several moments, experimenting with the position that best elongates the spine. Feel the wonderful stretch through the length of your back. Perform this stretch for 30 seconds before and after this exercise.

THE EXERCISE
Place your hands at the base of your skull, elbows extended. With your torso erect and your spine straight, inhale and slowly let the weight of your arms pull you toward the floor on a count of three . . . two . . . one. Exhale and slowly bring your elbows and torso up on a count of three . . . two . . . one, until your spine is straight and your head is aligned with your feet. Hold this position for one count. Repeat the prescribed number of repetitions. Stretch after each set by staying in the down or starting position.

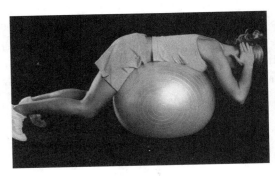 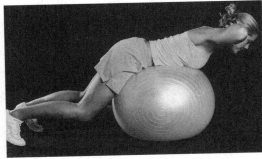

☆ Hollywood Pull-In

GET READY
Kneel on the floor and place your exercise ball directly in front of you. Lean your torso forward slightly, placing your forearms on the ball. Interlock your fingers. You are now in a position that approximates a bedtime prayer.

THE EXERCISE
Inhale and lean forward, pointing your hands forward as you go, allowing the ball to roll forward until it is between your elbows and wrists. Exhale and come back to the starting position. Inhale and repeat the prescribed number of repetitions. Stretch after each set using the back stretch.

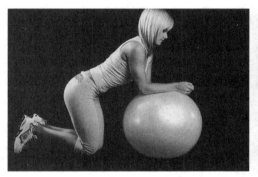 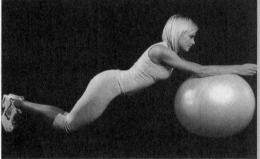

BACK STRETCH
Find a pole that is solid enough to support your weight. Facing the pole, place your feet on either side of its base. Interlock your fingers around the pole and place your hands above your head. Let the weight of your buttocks and torso fall away from the pole and allow your body to form the shape of an archer's bow. Feel the stretch between your shoulder blades and along the length of your back. Perform this stretch for 40 seconds after each set.

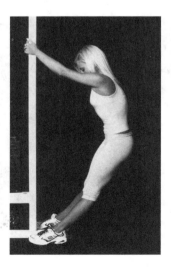

☆ Hollywood Shrug

The shrugs are ideal for working the trapezius muscles (traps), which are the muscles that connect the shoulders with the neck and the shoulder blades. For men, this exercise has two benefits. First, as seen from behind, developing the traps finishes the look of your back and complements the shoulder blades. Second, the weights effectively stretch these muscles and reduce tension. For women, developing the trapezius muscles gives the neck a longer and more elegant appearance. These muscles also accentuate the muscles of the shoulder blades, making backless dresses all the more flattering.

GET READY

Stand facing a mirror with your feet together. Your knees should not be locked but should be slightly bent. With a dumbbell in each hand, your palms should be facing your hips. Your back should be straight, and you should be looking directly in the eyes of your image in the mirror.

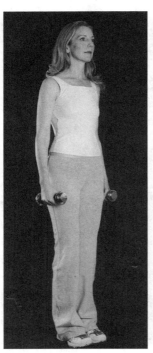
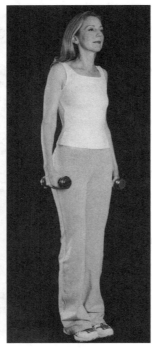

THE EXERCISE

Exhale and lift your shoulders toward your ears as if your body language could read: "I don't know." Hold for one count. Inhale and ease the dumbbells toward the floor on a count of three . . . two . . . one. Feel the stretch as you finish the inhalation. Exhale and repeat the prescribed number of repetitions. The stretch is built into this exercise, so rest for 15 seconds between each set.

Hollywood Shoulders

Think of your shoulders as the cherry on top of a sundae: without the cherry, it just isn't a sundae. Your shoulders are the key to completing your look. Development of these muscles will dramatically improve your posture and positively enhance the appearance of many other body parts.

There are three distinct areas of the deltoid or shoulder muscle: front, middle, and rear. Almost all of us have an overdeveloped front deltoid and an underdeveloped rear deltoid. Developing the rear deltoid will help pull your shoulders back, consequently lifting your chest, allowing the spine to become elongated, and enabling the abdominal muscles to better support your weight. In addition, the development of the rear deltoid will delineate where your shoulders end and the triceps begin, accentuate the bicep muscles, and best complement a total look for your arms and back.

Hollywood W Shoulders

The Hollywood W shoulders is an exercise of my own design, and it is tailored to work all three areas of the deltoid muscle. It is performed with a pair of dumbbells and is the most effective exercise for working the muscle to 100 percent of its ability. Even if you work out regularly, you will want to use fairly light weights for this exercise; this exercise will make you feel as if your shoulders are on fire.

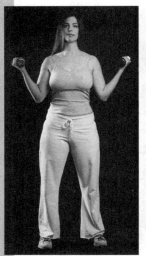 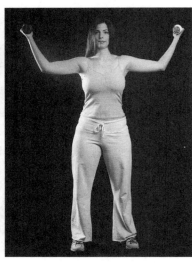

GET READY

With a dumbbell in each hand, stand up tall with your feet hip-width apart. With your palms facing front, bring the dumbbells to shoulder level, as if the weights were an extension of the shoulders. Your elbows should be pointed straight toward the floor. When you look in the mirror, you should be in the shape of a W.

THE EXERCISE

Exhale and drive your hands straight up toward the ceiling until the shape of your arms look likes a U or a goalpost. Hold this position for one count as you finish your exhalation. Inhale, and release back into the shape of a W on a count of three . . . two . . . one. Exhale and repeat for the prescribed number of repetitions. Stretch after each set using the shoulder stretch.

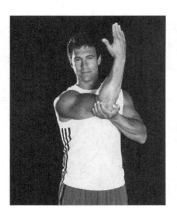

SHOULDER STRETCH

Standing up tall, extend your right arm straight out in front of you. Bend your elbow in a 90-degree angle, and turn your palm toward your face. Place your left hand on the right elbow and relax the right shoulder, letting it drop down. Use the left hand to gently hug the right arm to your chest. As you breathe in and out, allow this stretch to deepen. Maintain this stretch for at least 30 seconds before repeating on the left side.

⭐ Hollywood Twisting W

This is another unique exercise I have created to work all three areas of the deltoid muscles. It is performed with a pair of dumbbells and is effective for working the muscle to 100 percent of its ability. As you did in the W Shoulders, you will want to use fairly light weights for this exercise. This is another exercise that makes your shoulders feel like they are on fire.

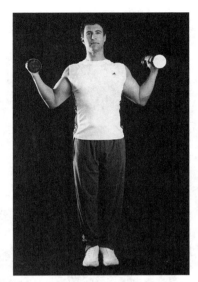

GET READY

With a dumbbell in each hand, stand up tall with your feet hip-width apart. With your palms facing front, bring the dumbbells to shoulder level, as if the weights were an extension of your shoulders. Your elbows should be pointed toward the floor. If you look in a mirror, you should be in the shape of a W.

THE EXERCISE

Exhale, and push the dumbbells up toward the ceiling, turning your wrists in a corkscrew-like motion until your arms are in the shape of a U and your palms are facing away from you. Hold for one count as you finish your exhalation. Release your arms back into the starting position on a count of three . . . two . . . one, turning your wrists back to their original position as you go. Perform the prescribed number of repetitions and stretch after each set using the shoulder stretch.

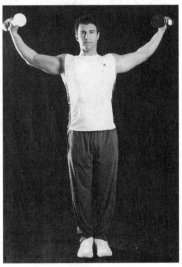

SHOULDER STRETCH

Standing up tall, extend your right arm straight out in front of you. Bend your elbow in a 90-degree angle, and turn your palm toward your face. Place your left hand on the right elbow and relax the right shoulder, letting it drop down (see photo on page 112). Use the left hand to gently hug the right arm to your chest. As you breathe in and out, allow this stretch to deepen. Maintain this stretch for at least 30 seconds before repeating on the left side.

☆ Hollywood Rear Delt

This is the most basic exercise for the rear portion of the deltoid. It is performed using two dumbbells. Low weight and proper technique are the keys.

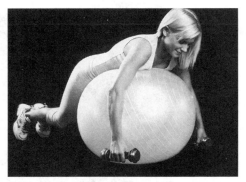

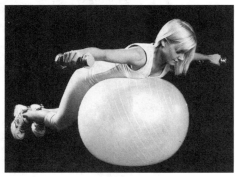

GET READY

With a dumbbell in each hand, kneel on the floor, and lower yourself onto your exercise ball so that it is against your lower chest and sternum. Push forward, let your knees come off the ground, and let your arms dangle straight down from your shoulders.

THE EXERCISE

Exhale, and leading with your elbows, lift the weights straight out to the sides so that your elbows are pointed toward the ceiling and the dumbbells are almost even with your shoulders. Inhale on a count of three . . . two . . . one, and bring the weights back down until they are in the starting position. Exhale, lock your elbows, and press the dumbbells back as far as you possibly can, squeezing the shoulder blades together and holding for a brief moment at the top of the movement as you finish your exhalation. Inhale and release back down into the starting position. (This is one repetition.) Complete the prescribed number of repetitions. Stretch after each set using the shoulder stretch.

SHOULDER STRETCH

Standing up tall, extend your right arm straight out in front of you. Bend your elbow in a 90-degree angle, and turn your palm toward your face. Place your left hand on the right elbow and relax the right shoulder, letting it drop down. Use the left hand to gently hug the right arm to your chest. As you breathe in and out, allow this stretch to deepen. Maintain this stretch for at least 30 seconds before repeating on the left side.

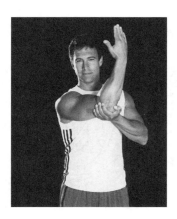

⭐ Hollywood Cheer

GET READY

With a dumbbell in each hand, stand with your feet planted firmly on the floor about hip-width apart. Bend your knees slightly so that they are not locked. The dumbbells are perpendicular to your body.

THE EXERCISE

This exercise is performed on a six-count. Exhale on a count of one and bring your arms up, knuckles toward the ceiling, until your arms are shoulder level and you are in the crucifix position. Hold for a moment as you finish your exhalation. Inhale on a count of two, and using only your shoulder joint, bring the heads of the dumbbells together in front of you (thumbs toward each other) until you are in the sleepwalking position. Exhale on a count of three, and on a count of four . . . five . . . six, reverse the steps until you are in the starting position. Perform the prescribed number of repetitions and stretch after each set using the shoulder stretch.

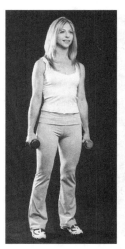 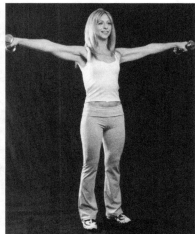 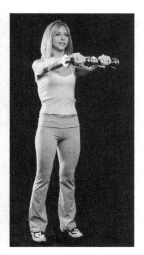

SHOULDER STRETCH

Standing up tall, extend your right arm straight out in front of you. Bend your elbow in a 90-degree angle, and turn your palm toward your face. Place your left hand on the right elbow and relax the right shoulder, letting it drop down (see photo on page 114). Use the left hand to gently hug the right arm to your chest. As you breathe in and out, allow this stretch to deepen. Maintain this stretch for at least 30 seconds before repeating on the left side.

☆ Hollywood Wings

Little wings are designed to completely exhaust the muscle to the point of fatigue. As your shoulder muscles reach this critical point, they will experience a significant burn. The range of motion is quite small here, and you will move the weights no more than 10 inches.

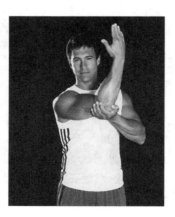

GET READY

Stand with a dumbbell in each hand. Plant your feet firmly on the floor shoulder-width apart. Raise your hands out to the sides until your arms are parallel to your shoulders and your knuckles are pointed toward the ceiling. Keeping your arms straight and your elbows locked, lower your arms 10 inches.

THE EXERCISE

Exhaling a puff of air, raise your arms toward the ceiling on a one count until your arms are just above your shoulders. Inhale and lower them 10 inches, on a count of two . . . three. Repeat the prescribed number of repetitions and stretch after each set using the shoulder stretch.

SHOULDER STRETCH

Standing up tall, extend your right arm straight out in front of you. Bend your elbow in a 90-degree angle, and turn your palm toward your face. Place your left hand on the right elbow and relax the right shoulder, letting it drop down. Use the left hand to gently hug the right arm to your chest. As you breathe in and out, allow this stretch to deepen. Maintain this stretch for at least 30 seconds before repeating on the left side.

Hollywood Wave

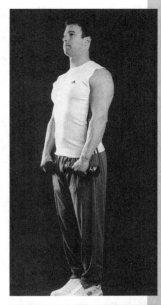

This exercise involves the entire shoulder, with an emphasis on the rear part of the deltoid to balance muscular strength.

GET READY

Stand with a dumbbell in each hand, with your feet together and your knees bent slightly. Position the dumbbells on your thighs, so that your knuckles are facing forward.

THE EXERCISE

Exhale, and leading with your knuckles, lift the dumbbells straight up in front of you until they are even with your shoulders and you are in the sleepwalking position. Leading with your elbows, bring the dumbbells straight back to your shoulders so that you are in a

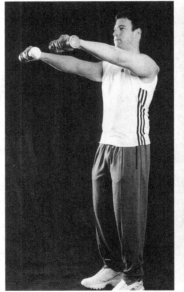

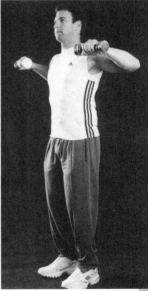

rowing position. Hold and finish your exhalation. Inhale and push the dumbbells straight out into the sleepwalking position. Release the dumbbells back down to the starting position on a count of three . . . two . . . one. Repeat the prescribed number of repetitions and stretch after each set using the shoulder stretch.

SHOULDER STRETCH

Standing up tall, extend your right arm straight out in front of you. Bend your elbow in a 90-degree angle, and turn your palm toward your face. Place your left hand on the right elbow and relax the right shoulder, letting it drop down (see photo on page 116). Use the left hand to gently hug the right arm to your chest. As you breathe in and out, allow this stretch to deepen. Maintain this stretch for at least 30 seconds before repeating on the left side.

Hollywood Chest

Your chest is a barometer of age. It is an indicator of firmness, fitness, and health. It is a key to attraction and sex appeal. For both men and women, it is a primary erogenous zone.

You are unique. Your look should be your own, and what you are striving for is the best that your individual body can be. The Hollywood look that is in right now has more to do with definition than size. Jennifer Lopez is not particularly well endowed, but she is extremely toned. Remember the infamous green dress she wore to the Grammys? Developing your chest in a very specific way can heighten your allure, regardless of your size.

Transforming your chest into the best that it can be is a three-part process. The following unique chest exercises have been designed to work in conjunction with the way in which the chest muscles are attached to your bones. The muscles of the chest have connection points at each shoulder, drape in a horseshoe or U shape, and attach along the length of the breastbone. Together each side of the chest forms a shape that would ideally look like a rounded W. To achieve a Hollywood chest, your primary objective will be to develop and define the edges of this muscle group. Then you will begin developing mass or filling in each horseshoe. The finishing touch will focus on building up the underdeveloped areas of this muscle group. These areas normally include the uppermost point where the muscle connects at the shoulder, the connection point alone the breastbone, and the highest points of each horseshoe along the collarbone.

By developing this muscle group, both men and women will achieve a finely toned chest that is as pleasing to the eye as it is to the touch. For women, this development may equate with the look of reconstructive surgery, lifting, separating, and firming the breasts, giving you a perkier, more sensual, and youthful-looking body.

Hollywood Fly

This exercise is designed to primarily work the inside and outside of the pectoral muscles. At the top of this exercise, I will ask you to squeeze your chest. You may ask, "Squeeze what?" In just a few short weeks, you will see and feel exactly what I am referring to. On either side of your breastbone, the musculature will develop, creating sort of a valley that rises up to each side of the chest. If the muscles in your chest were large and highly developed, you would actually be attempting to squeeze these muscles together.

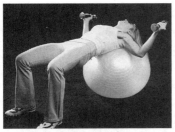

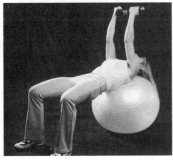

GET READY

With a dumbbell in each hand, position your exercise ball under the upper half of your back. Position your hands so that your knuckles are facing the ceiling, and bring your elbows down so that they are below you pointed toward the floor. Extend your arms to the side until they are almost fully extended. You should be feeling a deep stretch across your chest. Your arms stay in this position to start the exercise.

THE EXERCISE

Exhale and drive the weights up as if you were wrapping your arms over a barrel or a beach ball. When you are about halfway up, begin to straighten your arms and let the dumbbells come as close together as possible without touching as you reach the top of the movement. Hold this position for one count as you squeeze the chest muscles. Inhale and come down to the starting position on a count of three . . . two . . . one as you deepen the stretch across your chest. Really expose the chest. Do not bounce when you are in this position. Exhale and repeat for the prescribed number of repetitions. Stretch after each set using the chest stretch.

CHEST STRETCH

Find a pole or bar that is immovable and at least 6 feet tall, stand in a doorway, or lean against the end of a wall. With your right arm raised and at a 90-degree angle, place the forearm along this immovable object. Turn your torso away from your raised arm until you feel an incredible stretch across half of your chest. Hold this stretch for at least 30 seconds. Switch arms and perform this stretch on your left side for the same amount of time.

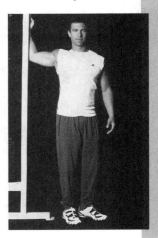

☆ Hollywood Incline Fly

Although this exercise is similar to the Hollywood fly, the angle of attack is changed to target the middle and uppermost regions of the pectoral muscles. To get the fullest possible benefit from this exercise, hold at the bottom of the movement and squeeze the chest muscles together at the top of the movement.

GET READY

With a dumbbell in each hand, sit down on your exercise ball. Roll down the ball so that it is positioned just below your shoulder blades and you are almost on a 45-degree angle. Plant your feet firmly on the floor with your legs a comfortable distance apart.

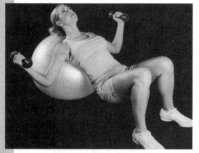

Bring the weights up so that your upper arms are at a 90-degree angle to your torso and the dumbbells are pointed in the same direction as your shoulders. Your upper arms are at a 90-degree angle with your forearms. Breathe in and allow the elbows to reach backward as you lower your hands until they are almost even with the middle of your chest. (If you were doing this exercise with a barbell, the bar would be just above your collarbone.) Feel the stretch across your upper chest.

THE EXERCISE

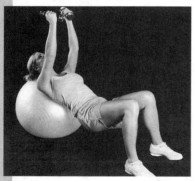

Exhale and drive the weights up as if you were wrapping your arms over a barrel or a beach ball. When you are about halfway up, begin to straighten your arms and let the dumbbells come as close together as possible without touching as you reach the top of the movement. Hold this position for one count as you squeeze the chest muscles. Inhale and come down to your starting position on a count of three . . . two . . . one as you deepen the stretch across your chest. Really expose the chest. Do not bounce when you are in this position. Exhale and repeat for the prescribed number of repetitions. Stretch after each set using the chest stretch.

CHEST STRETCH

Find a pole or bar that is immovable and at least 6 feet tall, stand in a doorway, or lean against the end of a wall. With your right arm raised and at a 90-degree angle, place the forearm along this immovable object (see photo on page 121). Turn your torso away from your raised arm until you feel an incredible stretch across half of your chest. Hold this stretch for at least 30 seconds. Switch arms and perform this stretch on your left side for the same amount of time.

Hollywood Decline Push-Up

This exercise works the uppermost portion of the pectoral muscles and is ideal for providing definition just under your collarbone.

GET READY

Drape yourself over your exercise ball. Place your hands on the floor and walk yourself forward until the exercise ball is under your knees. Situate yourself so that your hands are on the floor just wider than shoulder-width apart and you feel stabilized. Make sure

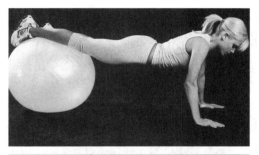

your legs are evenly spaced on either side of the exercise ball. You should be in the push-up position.

THE EXERCISE

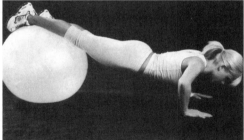

Inhale and slowly lower your chest toward the floor on a count of three . . . two . . . one. Hold at the bottom for a moment while you finish your inhalation. With an explosive motion, exhale and push yourself back up until your arms are straight and you have returned to your starting position. Hold at the top as you finish your exhalation. (As you become stronger and more advanced, move the ball toward your feet.) Repeat and perform the prescribed number of repetitions, stretching after each set using the chest stretch.

CHEST STRETCH

Find a pole or bar that is immovable and at least 6 feet tall, stand in a doorway, or lean against the end of a wall. With your right arm raised and at a 90-degree angle, place the forearm along this immovable object. Turn your torso away from your raised arm until you feel an incredible stretch across half of your chest. Hold this stretch for at least 30 seconds. Switch arms and perform this stretch on your left side for the same amount of time.

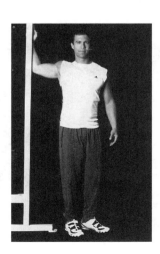

☆ Hollywood Frankenstein

This exercise is designed to work the upper third of your pectoral muscles and to enhance separation on either side of your sternum.

GET READY

Stand up tall with your feet about hip-width apart. Your legs should be straight but your knees should not be locked. Each hand should hold the head of one dumbbell. Let your arms relax.

THE EXERCISE

Exhale and slowly raise the dumbbell toward the ceiling on a one-count, until your arms are at shoulder level and you look like Frankenstein making an offering. Inhale and release the dumbbell back down to the starting position on a count of three ... two ... one. Repeat the prescribed number of repetitions and stretch after each set using the chest stretch.

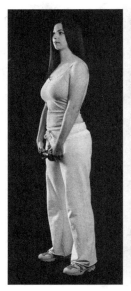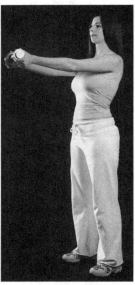

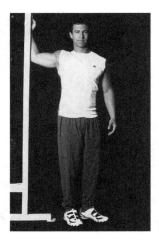

CHEST STRETCH

Find a pole or bar that is immovable and at least 6 feet tall, stand in a doorway, or lean against the end of a wall. With your right arm raised and at a 90-degree angle, place the forearm along this immovable object. Turn your torso away from your raised arm until you feel an incredible stretch across half of your chest. Hold this stretch for at least 30 seconds. Switch arms and perform this stretch on your left side for the same amount of time.

Hollywood C Sweep

This exercise is performed with dumbbells on the exercise ball and is designed to work the entire pectoral muscle. The basic movement is to trace a C around your torso with each hand. The key is to maximize the movement at the starting and ending points of the C sweep. The exercise begins with a deep stretch to hit the top of the pecs with pinpoint accuracy. Throughout the movement you will work the entire edge of the muscle. The exercise ends by flexing the chest muscles to develop their bottom portion.

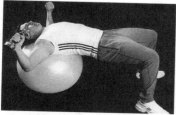

GET READY

With a dumbbell in each hand, lie back on your exercise ball, positioning the ball at the bottom of your shoulder blades. With your elbows pointed toward the ground, bring your hands slightly higher than the shoulders so that the dumbbells are even with your ears and your knuckles are facing the ceiling. You will now trace a C shape with each hand.

THE EXERCISE

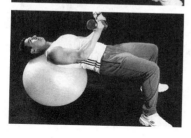

Exhale, and without raising your hands any higher, use the chest muscles to sweep the dumbbells to the level of your waist in the pattern of an arc. Continuing the exhalation and the arc-movement, gradually turn your wrists as your arms pass the waist, proceeding to trace the bottom of the C. During the last portion of this movement where you are finishing the C, raise your hands slightly. With the palms facing in the direction of your head, hold this position as you feel the bottom of the pectoral muscles flex. Inhale and reverse the C on a count of three . . . two . . . one. Feel the deep stretch across your chest as you finish your inhalation. Exhale and repeat the prescribed number of repetitions. Stretch after each set using the chest stretch.

CHEST STRETCH

Find a pole or bar that is immovable and at least 6 feet tall, stand in a doorway, or lean against the end of a wall. With your right arm raised and at a 90-degree angle, place the forearm along this immovable object (see photo on page 122). Turn your torso away from your raised arm until you feel an incredible stretch across half of your chest. Hold this stretch for at least 30 seconds. Switch arms and perform this stretch on your left side for the same amount of time.

⭐ Beginner Push-Up

THE EXERCISE

Lie facedown on the floor, preferably on a thick carpet or a mat. Cross your ankles, bend your knees, and lift your feet off the ground. Place your hands, palms down, just beyond your shoulders. Exhale and push your body away from the floor so that you are balancing on your hands and knees. Do not let the buttocks go too high, but rather let your body form a straight line from your knees to your head. Inhale and come down on a count of three . . . two . . . one until you almost touch the floor. Hold this position for one count as you finish your inhalation. Exhale and repeat for the prescribed number of repetitions. Stretch after each set using the chest stretch.

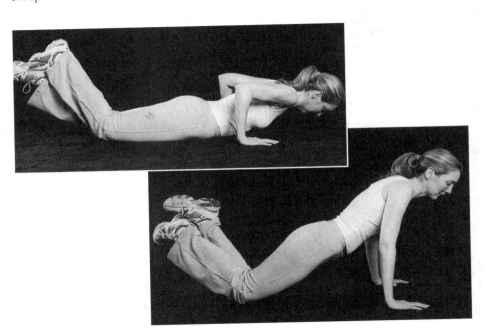

CHEST STRETCH

Find a pole or bar that is immovable and at least 6 feet tall, stand in a doorway, or lean against the end of a wall. With your right arm raised and at a 90-degree angle, place the forearm along this immovable object (see photo on page 125). Turn your torso away from your raised arm until you feel this incredible stretch across half of your chest. Hold this stretch for at least 30 seconds. Switch arms and perform this stretch on your left side for the same amount of time.

⭐ Advanced Push-Up

THE EXERCISE

Lie facedown on the floor. Curl your toes under your feet so that you are resting on the balls of your feet, and place your hands, palms down, just beyond your shoulders. Exhale and push away from the floor, keeping your body in a straight line from your head to your toes. Inhale and ease the body down on a count of three . . . two . . . one until your chest almost touches the floor. Hold this position for one count as you finish your inhalation. Exhale and repeat for the prescribed number of repetitions. Stretch after each set using the chest stretch.

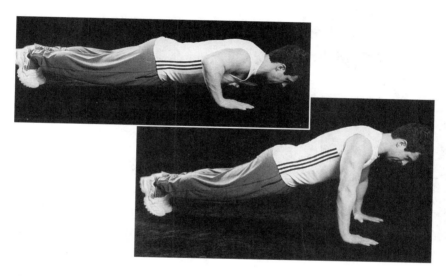

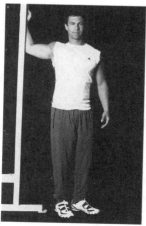

CHEST STRETCH

Find a pole or bar that is immovable and at least 6 feet tall, stand in a doorway, or lean against the end of a wall. With your right arm raised and at a 90-degree angle, place the forearm along this immovable object. Turn your torso away from your raised arm until you feel an incredible stretch across half of your chest. Hold this stretch for at least 30 seconds. Switch arms and perform this stretch on your left side for the same amount of time.

⭐ Hollywood Ball Push-Up

This exercise is an excellent way to determine if one pectoral muscle is stronger than the other, and it will help create symmetry and balance. It is an advanced exercise, so if it

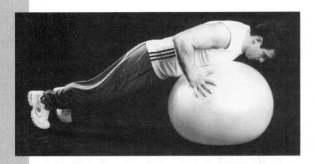

is too difficult right now, simply replace it with the Beginner Push Up (women) or the Advanced Push-Up (men). Try again the next time you see this exercise in your prescribed routine.

GET READY

Spread your legs just wider than shoulder-width apart as you drape yourself over your exercise ball. Your face should be pointed toward the floor. Walk yourself back carefully, allowing yourself to remain on top of the ball as it rolls toward your chin. When the ball is positioned in the middle of your chest, curl your toes under your feet so that you are resting on the balls of your feet. Place your hands on either side of the ball.

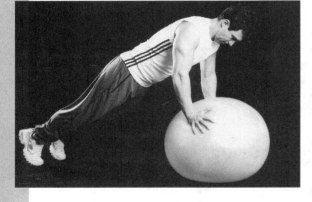

THE EXERCISE

Exhale and push away from the floor, keeping your body in a straight line from your head to your toes. Inhale and ease the body down on a count of three . . . two . . . one until your chest almost touches the ball. Hold this position for one count. Exhale and repeat for the prescribed number of repetitions. Stretch after each set using the chest stretch.

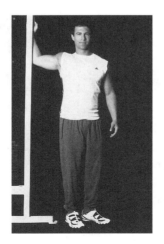

CHEST STRETCH

Find a pole or bar that is immovable and at least 6 feet tall, stand in a doorway, or lean against the end of a wall. With your right arm raised and at a 90-degree angle, place the forearm along this immovable object. Turn your torso away from your raised arm until you feel an incredible stretch across half of your chest. Hold this stretch for at least 30 seconds. Switch arms and perform this stretch on your left side for the same amount of time.

Hollywood Arms

For most men, the arms are a reflection of virility and machismo. For women, the arms symbolize an image and attitude that combines strength and femininity. Particularly for women, the arms are a common area of concern. Puffy biceps or flabby underarms are unflattering. Here's the good news: these muscles are some of the easiest to completely transform.

In Hollywood, bodybuilder bulk is no longer the rage. Today you will see definition, muscle separation or cut, and highly developed biceps and triceps. The sleeveless dresses of starlets on the red carpet, the love scenes of leading men, and the action pictures featuring favorite actors and actresses all highlight these symbols of strength.

There are two distinct areas that you will focus on when working your arms: the back of the arm (triceps) and the front area (biceps). Because we all lift many objects every day, our biceps are more developed than our triceps. To achieve a balance, make the triceps your primary focus. To create a stunning arm, you will work on improving the development, tone, and cut of the triceps. There is an altogether different strategy for developing your biceps. This particular muscle is simple in function: it can only contract. To prevent the formation of a short and tight muscle, you will spend as much time stretching this muscle as you do working it. The goal is to create beautifully elongated bicep muscles.

Hollywood Tricep Exercises

☆ Hollywood Tricep Extension

The tricep extension is designed to work all three areas of the muscle. The only portion of your body that will actually move is the elbow joint. Think of this joint as if it were a hinge on a door. The door does not wobble, and the wall does not weave back and forth; only the hinge moves.

GET READY

With a dumbbell in each hand, sit on top of your exercise ball so that you feel stable. Slowly walk your feet out, and lean back until you are lying back on the ball. Position the ball underneath your head and shoulder blades. Your feet should be a comfortable distance apart, planted firmly and flat against the floor for stability. Bring the dumbbells just above the very top of your forehead, and turn your wrists slightly so that the ends of the dumbbells nearest your head almost touch. Your elbows should be pointed toward the ceiling. Your thumbs should be nearest to your head, and the heels of your hands should be pointed away from your face. Bring your elbows close together so that they are no wider than shoulder-width apart.

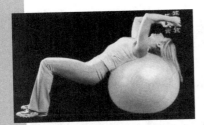

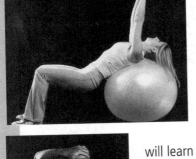

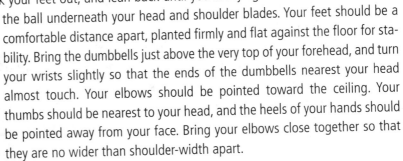

THE EXERCISE

Exhale and drive the weights up, turning your wrists so that your palms are pointed to the place where the wall meets the ceiling. Do not fully extend the arms, as it would take all the pressure off the triceps. Inhale on a count of three . . . two . . . one as you turn the wrists back to the starting position, and slowly bring the weights to the top of your forehead. This negative movement should remain very controlled. Come back too quickly and you will learn how this exercise got the nickname "brain crusher." Exhale and perform the prescribed number of repetitions. Stretch after each set using the tricep stretch.

TRICEP STRETCH

Either stand or sit at the end of a bench. Lift your right arm over your head and place your right hand between your shoulder blades. Place your left hand on your right elbow, and come as close as you can to pointing your elbow straight up toward the ceiling. Continue this stretch for at least 15 seconds. Repeat on the left side.

Hollywood Kickout

This exercise is designed to work both the inside and the outside of the tricep muscle, and it has been created to confuse the muscle with each repetition. It demands that the triceps be isolated, meaning that you will not swing your body to move the weight. Your elbows and wrists will be the only joints that actually move.

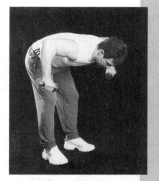

GET READY

With a dumbbell in each hand, stand with your feet slightly wider than hip-width apart. With your back straight and knees bent, lean forward until your torso is parallel with the ground. Raise your elbows until they are perpendicular to your torso, and bring the dumbbells to your chest with your palms facing toward you. You are now in the position of a football blocker. Using only your elbow hinge to move, release your forearms so that your arms are in a 90-degree angle and the dumbbells are perpendicular to your body.

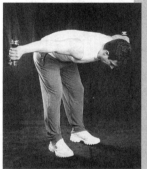

THE EXERCISE

Using only your elbow as a hinge, exhale and drive the weights out to the sides until your arms are fully extended. As you finish your exhalation, twist your wrists so that your palms are facing toward the floor. Twist back, inhale, and release back down to the starting position on a count of three . . . two . . . one.

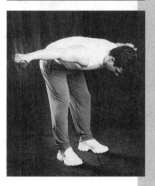

Exhale and drive the weights out to the sides until your arms are fully extended. As you finish your exhalation, twist your wrists so that your palms are facing toward the ceiling. Twist back, inhale, and release back down to the starting position on a count of three . . . two . . . one. Perform the prescribed number of repetitions, alternating the wrist twist on each rep. Stretch after each set using the tricep stretch.

TRICEP STRETCH

Either stand or sit at the end of a bench. Lift your right arm over your head and place your right hand between your shoulder blades. Place your left hand on your right elbow, and come as close as you can to pointing your elbow straight up toward the ceiling (see photo on page 128). Continue this stretch for at least 15 seconds. Repeat on the left side.

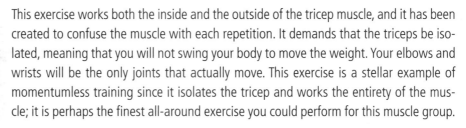

Hollywood Kickback

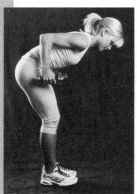

This exercise works both the inside and the outside of the tricep muscle, and it has been created to confuse the muscle with each repetition. It demands that the triceps be isolated, meaning that you will not swing your body to move the weight. Your elbows and wrists will be the only joints that actually move. This exercise is a stellar example of momentumless training since it isolates the tricep and works the entirety of the muscle; it is perhaps the finest all-around exercise you could perform for this muscle group.

GET READY

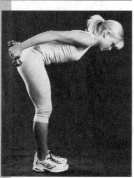

With a dumbbell in each hand, stand with your feet slightly wider than hip-width apart. With your back straight and knees bent, lean forward until your torso is parallel with the ground. Raise your elbows until they are parallel with your torso so that your arms are at a 90-degree angle and your knuckles are facing the floor. You are now in the position of a skier headed downhill. The basic movement in this exercise would be that used in propelling yourself downhill with ski poles. Press your upper arms tightly against the rib cage and do not let them move for the duration of the exercise. This will promote the isolation of the tricep muscles.

THE EXERCISE

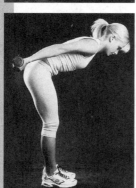

From this skiing position, use the elbows as hinges. Exhale and drive the weights behind you until your arms are fully extended. Hold this position for one count as you rotate your wrists so that your thumbs are facing each other and your palms are facing the ceiling. Finish your exhalation and rotate the wrists back to the neutral position. Inhale and slowly release your hands back to the starting position on a count of three . . . two . . . one.

Exhale to drive the weights back. Hold for one count. Turn the wrists so that your thumbs are pointing away from your body and your palms are facing the floor. Inhale to come back down to your starting point on a count of three . . . two . . . one. With each repetition, alternate between turning the wrists in and out. Repeat for the prescribed number of sets. Stretch after each set using the tricep stretch.

TRICEP STRETCH

Either stand or sit at the end of a bench. Lift your right arm over your head and place your right hand between your shoulder blades. Place your left hand on your right elbow, and come as close as you can to pointing your elbow straight up toward the ceiling (see photo on page 131). Continue this stretch for at least 15 seconds. Repeat on the left side.

Hollywood Ball Press

GET READY

Drape yourself over the exercise ball. Roll forward and place your hands, then your fore-arms, on the floor. Walk yourself forward until the ball is underneath your knees. Place your hands flat on the floor. Your forearms should be shoulder-width apart, parallel to your body.

THE EXERCISE

Exhale, and with an explosive movement, push up with your hands until your arms are fully extended. Hold as you finish your exhalation. Inhale, and using only your elbows as hinges, slowly lower yourself back down to the starting position on a count of three . . . two . . . one. Repeat for the prescribed number of repetitions. Stretch after each set using the tricep stretch.

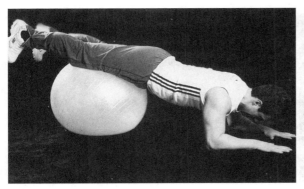
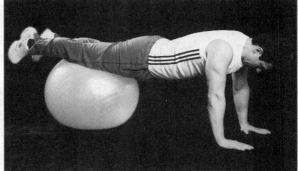

TRICEP STRETCH

Either stand or sit at the end of a bench. Lift your right arm over your head and place your right hand between your shoulder blades. Place your left hand on your right elbow, and come as close as you can to pointing your elbow straight up toward the ceiling. Continue this stretch for at least 15 seconds. Repeat on the left side.

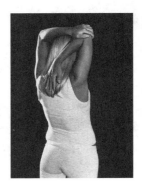

Hollywood Overhead Tri

The overhead tricep extension can be an awkward exercise. It is performed with dumbbells and is designed to totally isolate the tricep muscle. It is important not to be overly macho in choosing your weight. Start light on this exercise and work your way up over time.

GET READY

Stand up tall with your feet hip-width apart. With a dumbbell in your right hand, bring the weight directly behind your head and position the dumbbell so that it is parallel with your spine. Your right elbow should be pointed toward the ceiling, and your right bicep should be in a direct line with your right shoulder. The only joint that will move is your elbow. The shoulders, torso, and upper arms should remain in a fixed position throughout the exercise. The point is to isolate the triceps as much as possible.

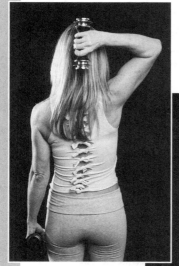

THE EXERCISE

Exhale and drive the weight up, extending your palms three-quarters of the way toward the ceiling. On the way up, the handle of the dumbbell should be in a direct line with your spine. Inhale and release the elbow joint back to the starting position on a count of three . . . two . . . one. Inhale and regroup as you feel the stretch.

Exhale and repeat for the specified number of repetitions. Switch to the left side and complete the specified number of repetitions, and you will have completed one set. Stretch the triceps after each set using the tricep stretch.

TRICEP STRETCH

Either stand or sit at the end of a bench. Lift your right arm over your head and place your right hand between your shoulder blades. Place your left hand on your right elbow, and come as close as you can to pointing your elbow straight up toward the ceiling (see photo on page 131). Continue this stretch for at least 15 seconds. Repeat on the left side.

⭐ Hollywood Dip

This exercise uses the weight of your body rather than weights to target all three areas of your triceps.

GET READY

You can use a bench, a ledge, or a sturdy chair.

LEDGE/BENCH   Sit on a flat ledge or bench with both of your legs on one side. Bring your hands close to your buttocks and grip the edge of the bench so that your elbows are pointing behind you.

CHAIR   Sit in the chair. Slide your buttocks forward until you almost slide off. Grasp the sides of the chair with each hand.

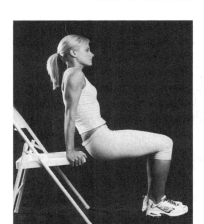

Position your feet about hip-width apart. Walk your feet out slightly and plant them firmly on the floor. Slide off the bench or chair until your legs are in a 90-degree angle and you are supporting your weight with your arms. Keep your back straight and your shoulders pressed down, and do not let your elbows point out to the sides.

THE EXERCISE

Inhale and lower your butt toward the floor on a count of three . . . two . . . one until your upper arms are parallel to the floor. Exhale and drive your body up, pressing your elbows toward each other to maintain their proper position. Straighten your arms until your elbows lock. Inhale and repeat for the prescribed number of repetitions. Stretch after each set using the tricep stretch.

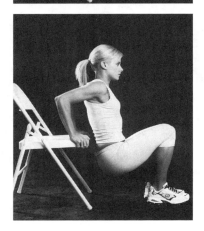

TRICEP STRETCH

Either stand or sit at the end of a bench. Lift your right arm over your head and place your right hand between your shoulder blades. Place your left hand on your right elbow, and come as close as you can to pointing your elbow straight up toward the ceiling (see photo on page 131). Continue this stretch for at least 15 seconds. Repeat on the left side.

Hollywood Bicep Exercises

⭐ Hollywood Squat Curl

The curl and the squat are the most basic leg and bicep exercises. Combined, you will discover that this particular exercise will take you into the aerobic and anaerobic levels rapidly. This exercise is performed with two dumbbells. There are two important factors to the movement. The first is correct elbow placement. Second, the bicep muscle must be isolated to ensure that only this muscle is involved in the movement of your arms.

GET READY

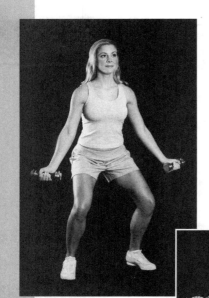

Your elbows should be at your sides, tucked into the ribs. Make certain that the elbows do not move from this fixed position. Do not swing the body to get the weights up. Use only the bicep muscles. When most people perform this exercise, they do not fully develop the entire muscle. You must make certain that you bring the weights all the way down so that you can totally stretch this muscle out. Failing to bring the weights down completely means that you are working only a small portion of the bicep, or about 35 percent of the entire muscle, making for an uneven, bulky, and malformed muscle. If you have proper technique, you can create a well-defined and elongated arm.

Stand up tall with a dumbbell in each hand, palms facing forward. Your feet should be slightly wider than shoulder-width apart, turned out slightly and planted firmly on the floor.

THE EXERCISE

Keeping your head and spine in alignment, inhale, bend your knees, and allow your butt to go back as if you were going to sit on a bench or chair on a count of three . . . two . . . one. Just as you would begin to make contact with the chair, exhale and drive up through the heels, simultaneously bringing the dumbbells up about three-quarters of the way toward your shoulders, turning your wrists so that the heels of your hands are pointing toward your chin. Straighten your legs, and hold this hand position for one count as you finish your exhalation and get the fullest possible contraction in the biceps.

Inhale and go down into your squat, releasing the weight all the way down on a count of three . . . two . . . one as your buttocks lower to sit on the imaginary chair. Feel the biceps stretch at the bottom of the exercise. Exhale while driving up and curling, turning the heels of your hands toward your chin as you finish your exhalation. Repeat for the prescribed number of repetitions. Stretch after each set using the bicep stretch.

BICEP STRETCH

Stand up tall in front of a mirror. Extend your arms straight out from your shoulders with your fingers pointing toward the ceiling as if you were standing in the middle of the street stopping traffic in both directions. With your elbows and hands locked in this position, rotate the arms so that your fingers are now pointing down. Lock your arms in this position and rotate only the wrists so that your hands are now in the traffic-stopping position. Hold for 20 seconds.

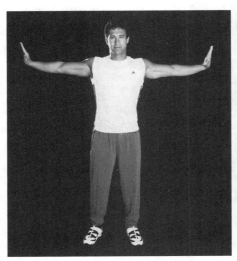 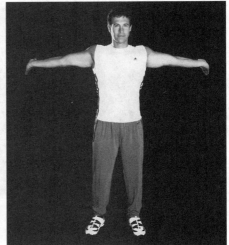

⭐ Hollywood Hammer Curl

The hammer curl is performed with a dumbbell in each hand. This exercise is designed to work the outside portion of the biceps and will have secondary benefits for the upper portion of your forearms.

GET READY

Stand up tall, arms at your sides, with a dumbbell in each hand so that your knuckles are facing the floor. Press your elbows into your torso, and keep them fixed throughout the exercise. This elbow placement will ensure the necessary isolation for the muscles you are working.

THE EXERCISE

Keeping the wrists and upper arms in a fixed position, exhale and bring both dumbbells three-quarters of the way toward the shoulders. The knuckles of the index fingers and

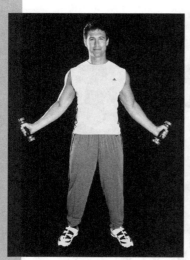 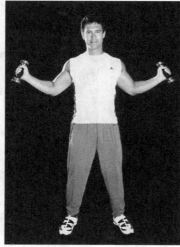

thumbs are now facing your shoulders, and you are in the position of a ready boxer. Hold for one count as you reach the top. Moving only with your elbow joints, inhale and release the dumbbells back down to the starting position on a count of three . . . two . . . one. Fully extend the arms to feel the stretch through your biceps. Repeat for the specified number of repetitions. Stretch after each set for at least 20 seconds using the bicep stretch.

BICEP STRETCH

Stand up tall in front of a mirror. Extend your arms straight out from your shoulders with your fingers pointing toward the ceiling as if you were standing in the middle of the street stopping traffic in both directions. With your elbows and hands locked in this position, rotate the arms so that your fingers are now pointing down. (See photos on page 135.) Lock your arms in this position and rotate only the wrists so that your hands are now in the traffic-stopping position. Hold for 20 seconds.

⭐ Hollywood Cross-Curl

I find this to be one of the most intense exercises for the biceps, and you just may find that it will exhaust your muscles.

GET READY

Hold a pair of dumbbells and stand tall with your spine straight and your head upright. Your feet should be about hip-width apart. With a dumbbell in each hand, extend your arms out to the sides in the crucifix position.

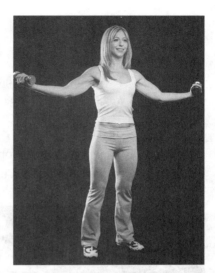

THE EXERCISE

Exhale and bring your fists three-quarters of the way toward your ears. Hold this position for one count as the biceps flex. Inhale and allow the hands to go back into the starting position on a count of three . . . two . . . one. Exhale and repeat for the prescribed number of repetitions, stretching with the bicep stretch after every set.

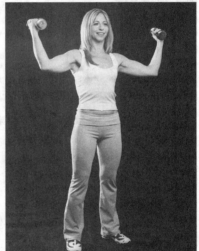

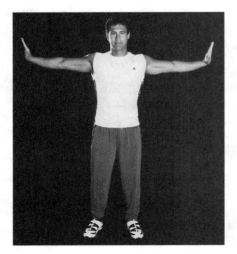

BICEP STRETCH

Stand up tall in front of a mirror. Extend your arms straight out from your shoulders with your fingers pointing toward the ceiling as if you were standing in the middle of the street stopping traffic in both directions. With your elbows and hands locked in this position, rotate the arms so that your fingers are now pointing down. Lock your arms in this position and rotate only the wrists so that your hands are now in the traffic-stopping position. Hold for 20 seconds.

⭐ Hollywood Ball Curl

This exercise is performed with two dumbbells and is ideal for completely isolating the biceps. You should get a full contraction from the entire bicep muscle. Do not swing the weights or use your back muscles to move the weights; isolation is the key to success.

GET READY

Drape yourself over your exercise ball. Position the ball so that it is at the top of your chest. Your arms should hang over the top, with your triceps resting against the ball. (If you are a woman and find this uncomfortable, position the ball just under your breasts and let your elbows rest against the ball.) Extend your arms fully and grip the dumbbells.

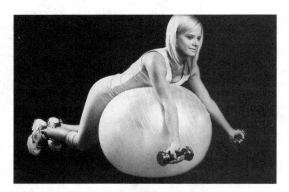

THE EXERCISE

Keeping your elbows in a fixed position, exhale and bring the weights up three-quarters of the way toward your head. When the weights reach this point, twist your wrists so that your thumbs are pointing away from you and the heels of your hands are turned toward your face. Finish your exhalation, holding this position for one count. Feel the entire biceps in full contraction. Inhale, and release the wrists and lower the weights on a count of three . . . two . . . one until your arms are fully extended. Feel the stretch throughout the biceps. Perform the designated number of repetitions. Stretch after each set for at least 20 seconds using the bicep stretch.

BICEP STRETCH

Stand up tall in front of a mirror. Extend your arms straight out from your shoulders with your fingers pointing toward the ceiling as if you were standing in the middle of the street stopping traffic in both directions. With your elbows and hands locked in this position, rotate the arms so that your fingers are now pointing down. (See photo on page 139.) Lock your arms in this position and rotate only the wrists so that your hands are now in the traffic-stopping position. Hold for 20 seconds.

⭐ Hollywood Karate Curl

GET READY

With a dumbbell in each hand, stand up tall with your feet hip-width apart.

THE EXERCISE

Sweep your right hand toward your left shoulder, then across your chest (passing below your chin) and into the curl position with an explosive motion on a count of one. (This move is typical of a martial arts block, a "ward off," or a parry.) Using only the hinge of your elbow, inhale, and slowly lower the dumbbell down into the starting position on a count of three…two . . . one. Turn your palms back toward your body, and repeat this exercise using your left arm. This is one rep. Perform the prescribed number of repetitions, and stretch after each set using the bicep stretch.

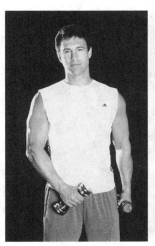 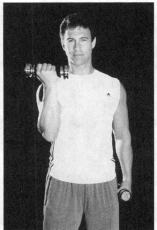 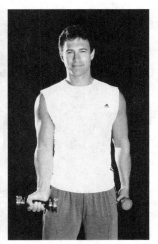

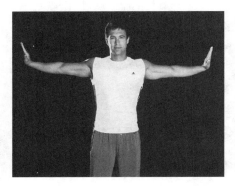

BICEP STRETCH

Stand up tall in front of a mirror. Extend your arms straight out from your shoulders with your fingers pointing toward the ceiling as if you were standing in the middle of the street stopping traffic in both directions. With your elbows and hands locked in this position, rotate the arms so that your fingers are now pointing down. Lock your arms in this position and rotate only the wrists so that your hands are now in the traffic-stopping position. Hold for 20 seconds.

Hollywood Abs

The ever-elusive Hollywood tummy is really a product of leanness rather than muscular definition. If you watch a Janet Jackson video, look at a film clip where the leading man takes off his shirt, or page through a magazine, you will see a washboard stomach. Rest assured, you have a similar washboard. Even people who are unable to move have these muscles. The difference is that most people have a layer of fat hiding them.

The goal is to decrease the amount of body fat and strengthen or develop this all-important area. By increasing the strength of your abdominal muscles, you can offset back problems or avoid them altogether. Strong abdominal muscles are necessary for proper posture and spinal alignment. Commonly called core muscles, they support the weight of your entire upper body. Strengthening this area will improve your spinal stability, providing you with a sense of buoyancy.

The muscles of the abdomen are a checkerboard of blocklike muscles that start underneath your rib cage and end where your torso connects with your thighs. There are also oblique muscles that stretch down each side of the abdomen.

The Hollywood ab routine will always be the last part of your workout because the abdominal muscles are the strongest of your core muscles. You must work this section of your body last to avoid muscular weakness and injuries in other parts of your body, especially your back. You will work the muscles by contracting them in many different directions and angles, then doing very specific exercises for the lower abdominals (below the belly button) and the obliques. To fully develop these muscles, you will never stretch them.

There is a very specific protocol for developing and strengthening the abdominal muscles. The lower abdominal muscles will come first in your ab routine. These muscles are generally weaker and are the most difficult to develop, so they will require extra attention. Then you will work the obliques or sides. Finally, you will work the middle and upper abdominal muscles simultaneously. For exercises that require you to be on the floor, I recommend using an exercise mat.

Hollywood Ball Crunch

GET READY

Drape yourself facedown over your exercise ball. Walk your hands forward until you are in a push-up position with the ball between your thighs and pelvic bone.

THE EXERCISE

Exhale, pull your belly button in toward your spine, and bring your knees toward your chest. Your buttocks will rise up and point toward the ceiling, and the ball will roll back between your shins and flexed feet. Inhale and release back down into your starting position on a count of three . . . two . . . one. Perform the prescribed number of repetitions.

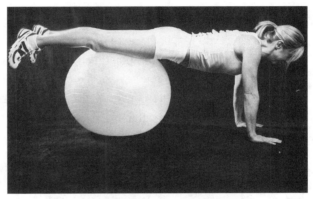

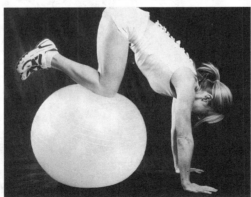

Hollywood Ball Small Sit-Up

This sit-up is performed while lying face up on your exercise ball. You should position the ball so that it is in the middle of your back, offering the greatest support for the lumbar area. You may perform this exercise with your fingers interlocked behind your head, your arms crossed on your chest with your hands on the opposite shoulders (the "I Dream of Jeannie" position), or by holding a dumbbell to your chest.

GET READY

Sit on top of the ball with your feet planted firmly on the floor a little more than hip-width apart. Roll down, moving your buttocks toward your feet, so that you have support for your lower back.

THE EXERCISE

Exhale, and keeping the spine and head straight, slowly raise your torso up on a count of one as far as you can, until you reach the point where you just begin to lose tension in the abdominal muscles. (This point marks the top of the motion.) Hold this position for a count of one. Inhale and release the torso back down a few inches. (This point marks the bottom of the movement.) Maintaining the abdominal contraction, perform the prescribed number of repetitions.

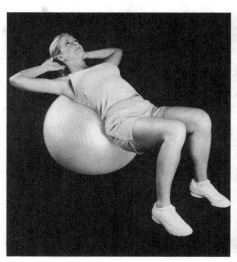 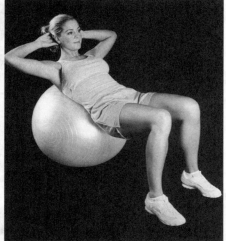

Hollywood Ball Pike

GET READY

Drape yourself facedown over your exercise ball. Walk your hands forward until you are in the push-up position with your knees resting on top of the ball.

THE EXERCISE

Exhale, and keeping your legs straight and your knees locked, pull your belly button in toward your spine, lifting your buttocks toward the ceiling on a count of one, until you are in an inverted V position. (In yoga, this would be similar to a "downward dog.") As you do this, the ball will roll back and be caught by your flexed feet. Finish your exhalation as you gently press your chest toward your knees. Inhale and slowly release back down into your starting position on a count of two . . . one. Perform the prescribed number of repetitions.

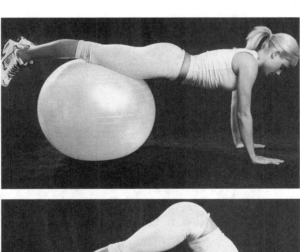

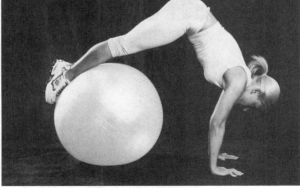

Hollywood Squeeze

GET READY

Lie down on the floor. Plant your feet on the ground with your knees pointed toward the ceiling. Place your exercise ball between your knees. Interlock your fingers and place your hands underneath your head.

THE EXERCISE

Exhale, pull your belly button into your spine, and squeeze the ball between your knees. Then simultaneously lift your shoulders off the ground and your hips off the floor, bringing your shoulders toward your knees and your knees toward your shoulders. Hold at the top of the movement to intensify the contraction, inhale, and release back down into the starting position and a count of two . . . one. As you become more advanced, try not to release all the way back down into the starting position, but only release as far as you can without losing the abdominal contraction. Repeat for the prescribed number of repetitions.

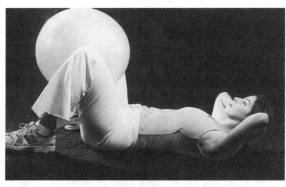

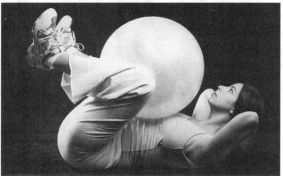

Hollywood Crunch

The crunch is just an improvement over the most basic form of sit-up. The goal is to bring your elbows to your knees. The key to getting the most abdominal work is to get the great majority of your hips off the ground as you fold your body. It is a fantastic overall abdominal muscle exercise and is even great for those with back problems. To minimize neck injuries, do not pull your head up with your hands—let your stomach muscles do the work. The point is to contract the abdominal muscles and not let them rest during the exercise. To keep the contraction going, perform these crunches as slowly as possible.

GET READY

Either place your hands underneath your head or cross your arms in front of you with your hands on the opposite shoulders. Begin with your head and feet on the floor.

THE EXERCISE

Exhale, simultaneously bringing your knees toward your elbows and lifting your hips and feet off the ground. Hold at the top of the crunch as you finish the exhalation. Slowly release and inhale, pulling your belly button in toward your spine as you unfold on a count of two . . . one. When you feel the point at which you lose the contraction, stop, inhale, and repeat for the prescribed number of repetitions.

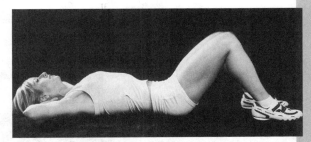

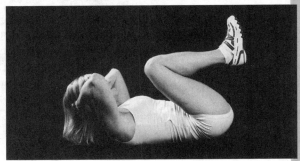

⭐ Hollywood Crossover Crunch

This exercise is like the Hollywood Crunch except your leg position is different. It is designed to strengthen all the areas of the abdominal group.

GET READY

Lie flat on your back with the soles of your feet on the floor and your knees pointed toward the ceiling. Cross your legs, placing the outside of your left ankle on top of your right knee. The crossed leg remains stationary throughout the exercise.

THE EXERCISE

Exhale and simultaneously bring your knees toward your elbows and lift your hips, feet, and shoulders off the ground, bringing your knees toward your elbows. Hold at the top of the crunch as you finish the exhalation. Inhale and come down on a count of two . . . one without letting your shoulder blades rest against the floor. Exhale and repeat for the prescribed number of repetitions. Repeat on the other side.

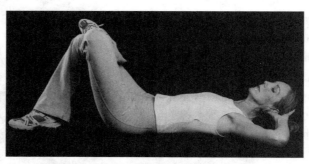

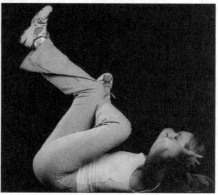

⭐ Hollywood Penguin

This exercise is designed to create strength and definition along the edges of the abdominal musculature and is fantastic for the oblique muscles. The point is to keep your shoulders and torso off the ground for the entire exercise.

GET READY

Lie flat on your back with your arms along your sides and your palms facing you. Bend your knees and bring your feet as close as you can to your buttocks. Place your feet flat on the floor so that your knees are pointed toward the ceiling. Exhale and pull your belly button into your spine. Maintain the contraction and inhale and tuck your chin into your chest, lifting your head, shoulders, and upper torso off the ground.

THE EXERCISE

Inhale and exhale evenly throughout the exercise. Touch your right hand to your right heel. Then touch your left hand to your left heel. Alternate between the right and the left quickly, and you will soon discover how this exercise was named.

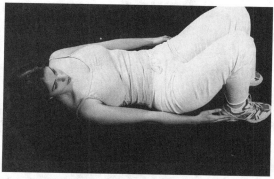

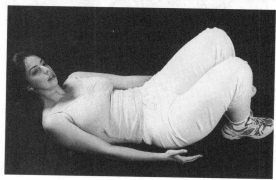

⭐Hollywood Leg Lift

To perform this exercise safely, find something very sturdy such as the legs of a heavy table, a pillar of some kind, or a very heavy chair.

GET READY

Lie on your back with your arms and legs fully extended. Grasp the heavy (or immovable) object with your hands. Lift your feet up until your body is shaped like an L.

THE EXERCISE

Exhale, pulling your belly button in toward your spine, and use your abdominal muscles to bring your buttocks off the ground. Lift your feet up toward the ceiling 6 to 10 inches on a one count, hold, and inhale. Release back down on a count of two . . . one. Repeat for the prescribed number of repetitions. As you become more advanced and your abdominal musculature becomes stronger, you may add ankle weights.

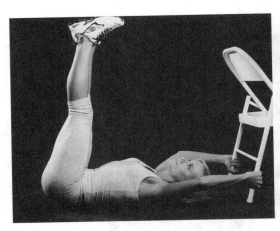 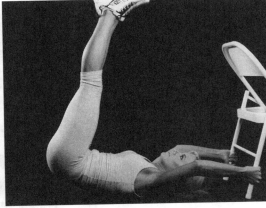

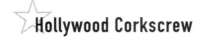
Hollywood Corkscrew

GET READY

Drape yourself facedown over your exercise ball. Walk your hands forward until you are in a push-up position with the ball between your ankles. Lock your elbows. Your upper body will remain fixed and rigid throughout this exercise. Your torso, abdomen, and legs will move from side to side as one unit. The movement is slow and steady. The more controlled this movement the greater the benefit.

THE EXERCISE

Exhale and pull your belly button into your spine. Maintain this contraction throughout the exercise. Inhale and allow the ball to roll slightly as your left foot lowers and your right hip lifts as much as it possibly can on a count of two . . . one. Exhale and come back into the starting position. Inhale and allow your right foot to lower and your left hip to lift as far as it possibly can on a count of two . . . one. This is one repetition. Repeat for the prescribed number of repetitions.

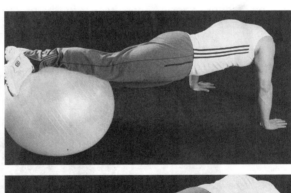

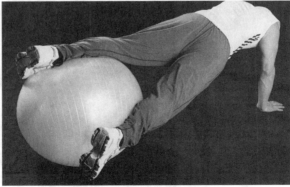

☆ Hollywood Side Raise

This exercise is performed using one heavy dumbbell of a challenging weight. The key is to stretch throughout the entire length of your torso, holding that stretch at the bottom of the movement.

GET READY

This is an excellent exercise to target the obliques. With a dumbbell in your right hand, stand up tall with your feet about hip-width apart. Turn your hand so that your palm is facing your hip. Place your left hand on your left hip.

THE EXERCISE

Exhale, and bending your waist to your right side, allow the dumbbell to lower toward the ground on a count of two . . . one. Keep your chest open and feel the stretch along your entire left side. Continue to stretch as much as you possibly can, maintaining the sensation that you are lengthening your spine. As you reach the maximum stretch, hold in this position and finish your exhalation. Inhale and come back to your starting position on a count of two . . . one. Repeat for the prescribed number of repetitions, then repeat on the other side.

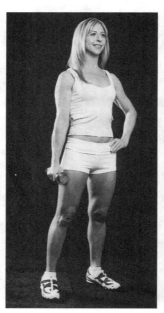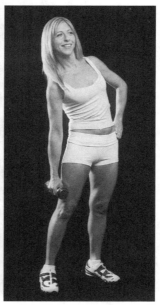

Hollywood Lying Side Raise

GET READY

Situate yourself on your exercise ball so that your left hip and torso are pressed against it and your hips are perpendicular to the floor. Your right foot should be behind the left foot as if you were taking a walking stride. Interlock your fingers and place them behind your head. Bend from the waist and allow your left elbow to drop down toward the floor. Feel the stretch along the entire length of the right side of your torso.

THE EXERCISE

Exhale, coming up to a position where your spine is in alignment. Continue your exhalation, coming up as far as you comfortably can. Inhale and drop the left elbow toward the floor on a count of two . . . one. Hold this position to feel the stretch. Exhale and repeat for the prescribed number of repetitions. Repeat on the other side.

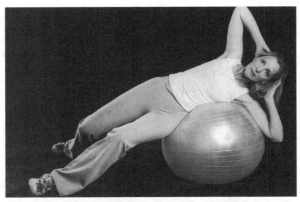

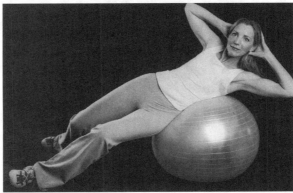

Completing Your Initiation

After this initiation phase, you will increase the duration and difficulty of your workouts so that you can experience dramatic results in the shortest possible time. I will teach you exactly what you need to do to reach your goals. You will create and adjust your own program. Just like every athlete I have ever trained, just like every celebrity who works out with me, just like every makeover story I have done in magazines or on television, you too can have a new lease on life and totally transform your body using the Hollywood body principles.

By the time you finish these first two weeks, you will have broken unhealthy eating cycles, short-circuited food addictions, established new habits of daily exercise, and eliminated 5 to 10 pounds of body fat. Every muscle in your body will have begun the process of a complete transformation. Not only will people begin to notice the difference in your appearance, but you might also become keenly aware that you feel completely different. You will experience a surge in your energy level. You will notice that your mindset is much more positive and upbeat. You might find yourself smiling or laughing more easily. You will sense a reduction in stress. You will begin to feel much more centered, capable, and ready for new challenges.

This new set of challenges is coming your way. Over the next four weeks, you will be on a program that is personalized for your specific needs. You are about to completely change the way your body looks.

What's Your
Hollywood Body Type?

Congratulations! In many ways, you have completed the most difficult portion of the process. You have begun. You are truly on a roll, so I do not want to break your rhythm with lengthy descriptions of what to do next and how to do it. I'll be as brief as possible so that you can maintain your momentum.

After completing the initiation, you are fit enough and prepared enough to do the work that will lead to dramatic physical changes. It is now time to get very specific about your personal needs, address those needs, and create a strategy that will allow you to look the way you want to look.

During the first two weeks of your initiation, the exercise and eating programs I designed for you were structured in a more generalized way to break unhealthy eating cycles and food addictions, raise your level of cardiovascular fitness, and begin the process of strengthening your muscles while familiarizing you with the revolutionary toning exercises. Over the next four weeks, the program I create for you will be much more specific to your personal needs.

Your needs are very much related to the way your body looks at this very moment. Over time, there has been a fascination with our physical differences. Beginning with the Greeks, much attention from the medical community has been paid to our varying shapes and sizes, and inferences for diagnoses have even been based on these categorizations. Throughout the twentieth century, physiologists studied our different shapes further, defined and categorized them, and even associated differing personality traits with each of these categories. Today, most professionals in the academic, scientific, medical, and health fields have adopted these categories of body shape classifications.

Within the health and fitness community, we generally use three categories for the human body: the ectomorph, the mesomorph, and the endomorph. We fashion or create specific training programs to suit these specific body types. Consequently, it is essential that you know your type so that you can follow the training regimen that best suits your personal needs.

The Ectomorph

Do you know people who can eat anything they want, never exercise, and are still thin? They are ectomorphs. Generally, an ectomorphic body is extremely lean. The ectomorph usually has a fragile, delicately built body and finds it difficult to gain weight or add muscle. With long limbs, small shoulders, and a lightly muscled physique, ectomorphs may appear taller than they really are. Ectomorphs are usually slight and small-boned, with a small chest and buttocks, giving them an almost linear physique.

Hollywood ectomorph bodies include Brad Pitt, Calista Flockhart, Tobey Maguire, Leelee Sobieski, Edward Norton, Steven Tyler (Aerosmith), Mick Jagger, Paris Hilton, models who are built like Kate Moss, and virtually every shooting guard and small forward in the NBA.

The Mesomorph

The mesomorph typically has an athletic, hard body and gains muscle easily. Endowed with excellent posture, thick skin, big bones, and mature muscle mass, the mesomorphic body is usually wider at the shoulders than at the hips. The male mesomorph will generally have a V or rectangular shape, whereas the female mesomorph will generally have a fairly chiseled hourglass figure.

Hollywood mesomorph bodies include Elizabeth Hurley, Sylvester Stallone, Jennifer Garner, Bruce Willis, Angela Bassett, Madonna, Arnold Schwarzenegger, and virtually every Mr. Universe.

The Endomorph

Like the mesomorph, the endomorph gains muscle easily; however, these muscles are generally underdeveloped, giving the endomorph a soft and round physique. Almost the polar opposite of the ectomorph, the endomorph gains weight easily and finds it difficult to eliminate excess body fat. This excess weight is generally carried around the belly (men) or on the hips (women). The endomorph generally has smaller shoulders, a high waist, and larger hips, sometimes leading to a pear-shaped physique.

Hollywood endomorph bodies include Jennifer Lopez, John Goodman, Kirstie Alley, Jack Black, Oprah Winfrey, and every offensive lineman in the NFL.

Reshaping Your Body Type

Most of us do not fit within these classic body types but have qualities of at least two. While you may or may not fit an exact definition, you have many qualities that are more akin to one of these prototypical bodies. Place yourself in one of the three categories so that you may create a program to reshape your body. It is time to take off your clothes and look in the mirror. What body type best fits your overall physique?

Over the next four weeks, the goal is to move away from the classic black-and-white definition of your body type into a gray area that is a more fitting blend of two body types. If you are more ectomorphic in appearance, the goal is to add muscle in strategic areas so that your appearance is more mesomorphic. If you are a true mesomorph, the goal is to become leaner and sculpt your musculature toward stunning definition so that you can look your absolute best. If you are more of an endomorph, the goal is to lean out the physique, creating muscle mass in specific areas so that women will move toward an hourglass figure and men will move toward a rectangular or tapered physique.

Bumps in the Road

After you have finished chapters 8 through 10, carefully read the opening of chapter 11 to better determine your next step. If you encounter any difficulty or face a challenge that is hard to navigate, don't quit! You need to get some support. Drop me a quick line at www.atighteru.com, and I will try to answer your question or help you with a solution.

8

Four Weeks to an Ectomorph Hollywood Body

The ectomorph is blessed with a very efficient metabolism. Everyone envies you. You probably burn off calories by sneezing. All your friends jokingly say that they hate you and wish they could be exactly like you. However, the grass is always greener on the other side. You know that having this physique is a blessing and a curse. Although you may eat almost anything you want, you know how difficult it is to add muscle or even to gain weight.

Generally, ectomorphs have shoulders that are approximately the width of their hips, giving the appearance of being thin, long, and wiry. Ectomorphs are quite linear, tubular, or cylindrical. If women gain weight, they will probably carry this weight below the belly button (known as the mound of Venus). Men may get a small paunch. Over the next four weeks, the goal is to eliminate any belly fat you may be carrying and create some curves to break up your linear appearance.

You will need to follow a very specific and rigid nutrition program, tone down cardiovascular exercise to the barest minimum for heart health, and structure your strength training regimen to add muscle and create as much size as you can.

Hollywood Nutrition for the Ectomorph

It is definitely time to move out of the initiation phase and eat your meals with a greater balance of carbohydrates and protein. If you are eating only five meals per day, add a sixth meal. Each of these meals must contain a significant portion of protein, since this additional protein will fuel your muscular growth. The size of your protein portion should approximate the size of your entire hand in length, width, and height. If you have difficulty ingesting this much protein, make certain your portion is at least the size of your palm and first knuckle.

Your carbohydrate choices may now include simple carbohydrates such as fruit, bread, rice, pasta, or potatoes, and the portion may be as large as your protein portion.

Hollywood Heart for the Ectomorph

You will stray from the initiation phase. Because you burn calories so efficiently, your cardiovascular exercise should be performed only for heart health. The Centers for Disease Control suggests a minimum of 25 to 30 minutes of exercise three days a week, which you should follow. Be conscious about what kind of exercise you perform, paying particular attention to your heart rate. Choose low-intensity exercise such as walking instead of jogging, aerobics, or a leisurely bike ride instead of a spinning class. Keep your heart rate at or below 70 percent of its maximum. Your three sessions can be at any time of the week, but make an effort to space them out evenly over the week.

Hollywood Sculpt for the Ectomorph

For both men and women, the goal of the workouts is to break up your linear qualities with some strategic curves. You need to create muscular density, size, and mass in some specific areas to give your body a more shapely appearance. If you look in the mirror today, you may indeed be very linear. After following my prescription for the next four weeks, you will begin to notice three distinct curves when you look head-on in the mirror. There will be a V from your shoulders to your waist, a slight bow from the lower hips to the knees, and another bow from the knees to the ankles. Increase your workout to four days per week, and on those days use fairly heavy weights. You will move that weight slowly and have fewer repetitions in each set.

The next four weeks of workouts for women begin on page 164. The goal of these workouts is to develop the shoulders, the lateral muscles, the deltoids, the upper legs, and the buttocks. By developing these muscle groups in the upper body, you will achieve a tapering effect from the (wider) shoulders down to the waist. Building size in your upper legs and buttocks will give your body more feminine curves.

The next four weeks of workouts for men begin on page 165. The goal of these workouts is to quickly provide you with a V shape. You will be working very hard to create size and bulk in your shoulders, deltoids, back, thighs, and calves. Use the heaviest weights you can move.

Supersets

On some days, you will utilize supersets. When a superset is prescribed, it indicates you are targeting two muscles or muscle groups. By using two exercises you will completely exhaust these muscles and stimulate particular muscles for growth and shape. When a superset is indicated, you will perform one set of exercise A, then a set of exercise B, and *then* stretch the muscle. For example, you might do one set of squat curls, then immediately perform one set of side kicks before stretching. By using alternating sets of two exercises, you will build size and shape in specific areas.

Perform three sets of ten repetitions. Stretch after each set.

WEEK ONE

DAY 1	Page	DAY 2	Page	DAY 3	Page	DAY 4	Page
Incline Fly	120	SUPERSET Rear Delt	114	Frankenstein	122	Side Kick	102
Beginner Push-Up	124	SUPERSET Wave	117	Beginner Push-Up	124	Inner Thigh	96
Pull-In	109	Ball Squat	98	Pull-Over	107	SUPERSET Kickout	129
Hyperextension	108	Arrow	95	Bent-Over Row	105	SUPERSET Tricep Extension	128
Hammer Curl	136	Overhead Tri	132	Squat Curl	134	W Shoulders	112
Ball Crunch	141	Leg Lift	148	Ball Pike	143	Ball Crunch	141
Crossover Crunch	146	Crunch	145	Side Raise	150	Lying Side Raise	151
Penguin	147	Ball Crunch	141	Ball Small Sit-Up	142	Ball Small Sit-Up	142

WEEK TWO

DAY 5	Page	DAY 6	Page	DAY 7	Page	DAY 8	Page
Fly	119	Lunge	93	Beginner Push-Up	124	SUPERSET Butt Lift	103
C Sweep	123	Leg Curl	97	Incline Fly	120	SUPERSET Reverse Lunge	94
Pull-In	109	Wings	116	Shrug	110	Calf Raise	99
One-Arm Row	106	SUPERSET Kickback	130	Ball Curl	138	Hyperextension	108
Karate Curl	139	SUPERSET Dip	133	Squat Curl	134	Cross-Curl	137
Squeeze	144	Leg Lift	148	Ball Pike	143	Crossover Crunch	146
Lying Side Raise	151	Side Raise	150	Lying Side Raise	151	Penguin	147
Ball Small Sit-Up	142	Penguin	147	Crunch	145	Ball Small Sit-Up	142

WEEK THREE

DAY 9	Page	DAY 10	Page	DAY 11	Page	DAY 12	Page
Incline Fly	120	Ball Lunge	101	SUPERSET Tricep Extension	128	Bent-Over Row	105
Frankenstein	122	Arrow	95	SUPERSET Overhead Tri	132	Pull-Over	107
Cheer	115	One-Arm Row	106	Rear Delt	114	Squat Curl	134
Twisting W	113	Pull-In	109	W Shoulders	112	Leg Curl	97
Ball Press	131	Hammer Curl	136	C Sweep	123	Side Kick	102
Ball Crunch	141	Leg Lift	148	Corkscrew	149	Inner Thigh	96
Corkscrew	149	Lying Side Raise	151	Ball Pike	143	Crossover Crunch	146
Side Raise	150	Squeeze	144	Ball Small Sit-Up	142	Crunch	145
						Penguin	147

DAY 13	Page	DAY 14	Page	DAY 15	Page	DAY 16	Page
Wave	117	Shrug	110	Incline Fly	120	Lunge	93
Wings	116	One-Arm Row	106	Ball Push-Up	126	Side Kick	102
Decline Push-Up	121	Karate Curl	139	Twisting W	113	Arrow	95
Kickout	129	Butt Lift	103	Frankenstein	122	Pull-In	109
Dip	133	Ball Squat	98	Kickback	130	Ball Curl	138
Ball Crunch	141	Corkscrew	149	Ball Pike	143	Crunch	145
Leg Lift	148	Side Raise	150	Penguin	147	Lying Side Raise	151
Squeeze	144	Ball Small Sit-Up	142	Crossover Crunch	146	Ball Small Sit-Up	142

SHAPING AND SCULPTING WORKOUTS FOR THE MALE ECTOMORPH

Perform three sets of ten repetitions. Stretch after each set.

WEEK ONE

DAY 1	Page	DAY 2	Page	DAY 3	Page	DAY 4	Page
Fly	119	Ball Squat	98	Tricep Extension	128	Ball Lunge	101
Decline Push-Up	121	Leg Curl	97	Kickback	130	Calf Raise	99
W Shoulders	112	Lunge	93	Incline Fly	120	One-Arm Row	106
Frankenstein	122	Bent-Over Row	105	Frankenstein	122	Pull-Over	107
Dip	133	Karate Curl	139	Twisting W	113	Ball Curl	138
Leg Lift	148	Ball Crunch	141	Crossover Crunch	146	Ball Pike	143
Crunch	145	Corkscrew	149	Squeeze	144	Side Raise	150
Penguin	147	Ball Small Sit-Up	142	Lying Side Raise	151	Ball Small Sit-Up	142

WEEK TWO

DAY 5	Page	DAY 6	Page	DAY 7	Page	DAY 8	Page
C Sweep	123	Reverse Lunge	94	Wave	117	Bent-Over Row	105
Rear Delt	114	Arrow	95	Ball Push-Up	126	Shrug	110
Wings	116	Squat Curl	134	Fly	119	Hammer Curl	136
Kickout	129	Pull-In	109	Overhead Tri	132	Karate Curl	139
Ball Press	131	Hyperextension	108	Dip	133	Leg Curl	97
Leg Lift	148	Ball Crunch	141	Leg Lift	148	Ball Pike	143
Penguin	147	Lying Side Raise	151	Corkscrew	149	Penguin	147
Crunch	145	Squeeze	144	Squeeze	144	Crunch	145

DAY 9	Page	DAY 10	Page	DAY 11	Page	DAY 12	Page
C Sweep	123	Ball Lunge	101	Decline Push-Up	121	Ball Squat	98
Advanced Push-Up	125	Reverse Lunge	94	Frankenstein	122	Leg Curl	97
W Shoulders	112	One-Arm Row	106	Twisting W	113	Pull-In	109
Cheer	115	Pull-Over	107	Kickback	130	Karate Curl	139
Tricep Extension	128	Ball Curl	138	Ball Press	131	Crunch	145
Crossover Crunch	146	Ball Crunch	141	Squeeze	144	Corkscrew	149
Side Raise	150	Lying Side Raise	151	Crunch	145	Ball Small Sit-Up	142
Squeeze	144	Ball Small Sit-Up	142	Penguin	147		

DAY 13	Page	DAY 14	Page	DAY 15	Page	DAY 16	Page
Kickout	129	Ball Squat	98	W Shoulders	112	One-Arm Row	106
Wings	116	Leg Curl	97	Decline Push-Up	121	Pull-Over	107
Rear Delt	114	Pull-In	109	C Sweep	123	Hammer Curl	136
Ball Push-Up	126	Karate Curl	139	Overhead Tri	132	Squat Curl	134
Incline Fly	120	Ball Curl	138	Kickback	130	Calf Raise	99
Leg Lift	148	Crossover Crunch	146	Squeeze	144	Ball Crunch	141
Ball Pike	143	Penguin	147	Lying Side Raise	151	Corkscrew	149
Squeeze	144	Ball Small Sit-Up	142	Crunch	145	Side Raise	150

9

Four Weeks to a Mesomorph Hollywood Body

If you have a mesomorphic body, you are indeed quite lucky. The physique you have been endowed with has provided you with a very nice foundation from which to work. Because the mesomorph is able to gain muscle mass quickly and is typically wider at the shoulders than at the hips, the possibilities for creating outstanding definition and shape are almost limitless. If you gain fat, your thick frame enables you to disguise it better than most people; however, if you do gain weight, it tends to gather around or above your belt line, giving you a "spare tire" emphasis.

Your toning program focuses on reducing your waistline, then simply shaping and contouring what you already have. The goal is to create a lot of shape. For women, the ideal is to have a very taut and chiseled hourglass figure. For men, the goal is to achieve a tapered physique. You are going to slowly alter your nutrition program, increase the intensity and perhaps the length of your cardiovascular workouts, and mix heavy strength-training days to stimulate muscular growth with light days to create tone.

Hollywood Nutrition for the Mesomorph

You are predisposed to gain muscle easily, so simply follow my prescription for toning and shaping and let nature take its course. The goal is to slenderize your body so that you can see the magic happen. You must keep your eating under control.

During the initiation, you set up new eating habits and did away with most of the poor ones. Be especially vigilant about the protein and carbohydrate choices on page 37. For the next month, try to limit your food choices to primary choices. Allow yourself to eat secondary carbohydrate choices one day per week, but make sure to adhere to the appropriate ratios. This will help you avoid uncontrollable carbohydrate cravings.

Hollywood Heart for the Mesomorph

Since the primary focus is to become more lean, increase the intensity and duration of your cardiovascular workouts. You will be exercising more intensely five days per week (rather than six). During your first week postinitiation, exercise for at least 30 minutes, striving to keep your heart rate between 70 and 80 percent of your maximum. During the second week, increase the duration of these sessions by 5 minutes. In week three, increase the duration of the session by another 5 minutes, and during each session insert three 2-minute bursts where you take your heart rate to 85 percent of your maximum. In week four, do not increase the duration of your cardiovascular session, but do try the interval training system (see page 200). You will exercise for specific blocks of time, alternating between a pace where your heart rate is in the 70 percent range and an interval where you sustain a heart rate in the 85 to 90 percent range. One day you will do a 2-minute interval, the next day you will do a 3-minute interval, and you will continue to alternate between the two so that you can achieve greater results by constantly surprising your body.

Hollywood Sculpt for the Mesomorph

The only downside of having a mesomorphic body is that you are thickly muscled. This thickness is especially noticeable in your waist. Although you can become lean, most mesomorphs will never be truly thin. You need to consciously shape and tone your muscles as a sort of camouflage to give the appearance of thinness. You will pay particular attention to specific areas of muscular development to create a tapered line from your shoulders to your hips.

Your program is designed specifically to be a total-body workout. Each time you tone, you will work every muscle group in your body. You will target specific areas and attempt to get the cut or definition described in chapter 5. You will also target the lateral muscles, shoulders, and deltoids to provide a tapering effect and to "lower" your waist.

Women will notice a great deal of shapeliness over the next four weeks. Your workouts are detailed on page 173. The objective is to further accentuate a full hourglass figure. You will strive to shape and contour your physique. Begin by strength training three days per week. Alternate between heavy and light days. On heavy days, move more weight and use fewer repetitions to stimulate muscular growth. On light days, move less weight but do many more repetitions to cut, tone, and shape the muscular structure.

For men, the secret to success depends on your ability to decrease the size of your inner tube and/or love handles. Your waist will probably never be much smaller than 32 inches. But when your body fat drops below 15 percent, you will see some amazing changes to your physique. You will be creating a very definite shape, and these workouts are all laid out for you on page 174.

Over these next four weeks, you will consciously strive to create a tapered physique. While your exercise regimen has been designed as a total-body workout to define and cut the musculature in the most flattering way, you will concentrate on creating a chiseled V from your shoulders to your hips.

Supersets

On some days, you will utilize supersets. When a superset is prescribed, it indicates you are targeting two muscles or muscle groups. By using two exercises you will completely exhaust these muscles and stimulate particular muscles for growth and shape. When a superset is indicated, you will perform one set of exercise A, then a set of exercise B, and *then* stretch the muscle. For example, you might do one set of squat curls, then immediately perform one set of side kicks before stretching. By using alternating sets of two exercises, you will build size and shape in specific areas.

Giant Sets

A giant set combines three exercises to build stamina and to make you work out to an anerobic level. When indicated, you will perform one set of exercise A, immediately followed by exercise B, then a set of exercise C, before stretching the muscle out. For instance, you might perform a set of beginner push-ups, immediately followed by a set of W shoulders, immediately followed by a set of ball curls, and *then* stretch the muscles out. By using combinations of exercises to target certain muscles, you will stimulate the greatest possible results in the quickest possible time.

SHAPING AND SCULPTING WORKOUTS FOR THE FEMALE MESOMORPH

Perform two sets of fifteen repetitions. Stretch after each set or superset.

WEEK ONE

DAY 1 (light)	Page	DAY 2 (heavy)	Page	DAY 3 (light)	Page
Fly	119	Side Kick	102	One-Arm Row	106
Kickback	130	Butt Lift	103	Rear Delt	114
Bent-Over Row	105	Beginner Push-Up	124	Ball Squat	98
Squat Curl	134	Dip	133	Arrow	95
W Shoulders	112	Wings	116	C Sweep	123
Crunch	145	Cross-Curl	137	Karate Curl	139
Leg Lift	148	Ball Crunch	141	Corkscrew	149
Ball Small Sit-Up	142	Lying Side Raise	151	Ball Crunch	141
		Squeeze	144	Ball Small Sit-Up	142

WEEK TWO

DAY 4 (heavy)	Page	DAY 5 (light)	Page	DAY 6 (heavy)	Page
Twisting W	113	Reverse Lunge	94	Incline Fly	120
Frankenstein	122	Butt Lift	103	Ball Press	131
Overhead Tri	132	Pull-Over	107	Hyperextension	108
Pull-In	109	Wave	117	Shrug	110
Ball Curl	138	Cross-Curl	137	Inner Thigh	96
Lunge	93	Tricep Extension	128	Leg Curl	97
Corkscrew	149	Leg Lift	148	Ball Pike	143
Ball Crunch	141	Lying Side Raise	151	Side Raise	150
Ball Small Sit-Up	142	Crunch	145	Squeeze	144

WEEK THREE

DAY 7 (light)	Page	DAY 8 (heavy)	Page	DAY 9 (light)	Page
Ball Lunge	101	Decline Push-Up	121	Inner Thigh	96
Side Kick	102	Rear Delt	114	Butt Lift	103
Ball Push-Up	126	Bent-Over Row	105	Calf Raise	99
Kickback	130	Squat Curl	134	Dip	133
Wings	116	Arrow	95	Fly	119
Hammer Curl	136	Leg Curl	97	One-Arm Row	106
Ball Crunch	138	Crossover Crunch	146	Cross-Curl	137
Penguin	147	Lying Side Raise	151	Corkscrew	149
Side Raise	150	Crunch	145	Ball Pike	143
				Penguin	147

WEEK FOUR

DAY 10 (heavy)	Page	DAY 11 (light)	Page	DAY 12 (heavy)	Page
SUPERSET Ball Squat	98	Pull-In	109	SUPERSET Arrow	95
SUPERSET Side Kick	102	Pull-Over	107	SUPERSET Butt Lift	103
SUPERSET Wave	117	SUPERSET Ball Curl	138	SUPERSET C Sweep	123
SUPERSET Karate Curl	139	SUPERSET Incline Fly	120	SUPERSET Overhead Tri	132
Frankenstein	122	Tricep Extension	128	SUPERSET Twisting W	113
Kickout	129	Reverse Lunge	94	SUPERSET Hammer Curl	136
Squeeze	144	Leg Lift	148	Ball Pike	143
Ball Crunch	141	Side Raise	150	Corkscrew	149
Ball Small Sit-Up	142	Crossover Crunch	146	Lying Side Raise	151

SHAPING AND SCULPTING WORKOUTS FOR THE MALE MESOMORPH

Perform two sets of fifteen repetitions. Stretch after each set, superset, or giant set.

WEEK ONE

DAY 1 (light)	Page	DAY 2 (heavy)	Page	DAY 3 (light)	Page
SUPERSET Ball Lunge	101	SUPERSET One-Arm Row	106	Ball Push-Up	126
SUPERSET Lunge	93	SUPERSET Hyperextension	108	Incline Fly	120
SUPERSET Decline Push-Up	121	Squat Curl	134	SUPERSET Rear Delt	114
SUPERSET Kickback	130	Leg Curl	97	SUPERSET Ball Curl	138
W Shoulders	112	SUPERSET Ball Press	131	Pull-Over	107
Karate Curl	139	SUPERSET C Sweep	123	Dip	133
Ball Crunch	141	Corkscrew	149	Crunch	145
Leg Lift	148	Squeeze	144	Crossover Crunch	146
Side Raise	150	Penguin	147	Lying Side Raise	151

WEEK TWO

DAY 4 (heavy)	Page	DAY 5 (light)	Page	DAY 6 (heavy)	Page
Ball Squat	98	SUPERSET Fly	119	Pull-In	109
Arrow	95	SUPERSET Overhead Tri	132	SUPERSET Bent-Over Row	105
SUPERSET Twisting W	113	Advanced Push-Up	125	SUPERSET Cheer	115
SUPERSET Wings	116	Wave	117	Frankenstein	122
SUPERSET Tricep Extension	128	Reverse Lunge	94	Kickout	129
SUPERSET Hammer Curl	136	Squat Curl	134	Calf Raise	99
Squeeze	144	Ball Pike	143	Crunch	145
Leg Lift	148	Penguin	147	Leg Lift	148
Corkscrew	149	Ball Small Sit-Up	142	Lying Side Raise	151

WEEK THREE

DAY 7 (light)	Page	DAY 8 (heavy)	Page	DAY 9 (light)	Page
Leg Curl	97	One-Arm Row	106	Incline Fly	120
Lunge	93	C Sweep	123	Ball Push-Up	126
SUPERSET Decline Push-Up	121	*SUPERSET* Rear Delt	114	*SUPERSET* Dip	133
SUPERSET Ball Press	131	*SUPERSET* Kickback	130	*SUPERSET* Twisting W	113
SUPERSET W Shoulders	112	Ball Lunge	101	Pull-Over	107
SUPERSET Karate Curl	139	Cross-Curl	137	Reverse Lunge	94
Ball Crunch	141	Ball Pike	143	Calf Raise	99
Side Raise	150	Crunch	145	Leg Lift	148
Squeeze	144	Ball Small Sit-Up	142	Leg Curl	97
				Corkscrew	149

WEEK FOUR

DAY 10 (heavy)	Page	DAY 11 (light)	Page	DAY 12 (heavy)	Page
Ball Squat	98	*SUPERSET* Wings	116	Arrow	95
SUPERSET Fly	119	*SUPERSET* Wave	117	Lunge	93
SUPERSET Tricep Extension	128	Overhead Tri	132	*GIANT SET* One-Arm Row	106
GIANT SET Shrug	110	Frankenstein	122	*GIANT SET* Shrug	110
GIANT SET Pull-In	109	Bent-Over Row	105	*GIANT SET* Kickout	129
GIANT SET Ball Curl	138	Squat Curl	134	Karate Curl	139
Crunch	145	Ball Pike	143	Leg Lift	148
Squeeze	144	Ball Crunch	141	Corkscrew	149
Side Raise	150	Side Raise	150	Ball Small Sit-Up	142

10

Four Weeks to
an Endomorph
Hollywood Body

If you are a true endomorph, I do not have to tell you how difficult it is to lose weight or make dramatic changes to your appearance. You will never look like Paris Hilton or Edward Norton. Even wanting to look like these people is destructive because it is an unattainable goal. The trick, however, is to whittle away at your present physique and melt enough body fat to become more of a mesomorph.

Not all endomorphs look like NFL linemen. Take a close look at Oprah today and compare this look with her 1995 look—there is a big difference. Check out Jennifer Lopez. There are some very fit, high-profile endomorphs out there.

I have had many endomorph clients. For whatever reason, people who fit within this group are predominantly women. When I first meet them for a consultation, most endomorphs are truly puzzled by their bodies, feeling that they are one body type above the belly button and quite another type below. In fact, there are some significant challenges for the endomorphic physique, and many of these challenges stem from addressing the upper and lower halves of the body while maintaining an all-inclusive program. For you, this physical transformation is going to be a process.

The good news is you have already begun. Just by completing the initiation, you have made great strides to create the foundation for your transformation. You have set up excellent eating and exercise habits. This will be the focus of your work for the next four weeks. Your goal is to continue the process of shrinking your fat cells. You will begin to structure your toning workouts to develop muscle groups that will create balance for your hips. The focus of these new workout sessions will be on your shoulders and back. The objective is to become an ectomorph/mesomorph combination. Women will strive to contour their physiques into hourglass figures, and men will sculpt their bodies to appear more rectangular or square.

Hollywood Nutrition for the Endomorph

You have done some terrific work over the last two weeks to break unhealthy habits and create a new metabolic rhythm. In moving forward, it may be necessary to experiment with your nutritional program so that you experience greater results. If you haven't already done so, find out your body fat percentage.

For the next two weeks, continue doing exactly what you have been doing but with one significant exception. Your protein portion should still be no larger than the height, length, and width of your palm; however, your protein choices may now include secondary options. If you choose a secondary protein choice, you must adjust your carbohydrate portion accordingly (see page 35). Continue to refrain from secondary carbohydrate choices, but allow yourself one day a week for a secondary choice so that your body does not develop cravings. Make sensible choices, and combine these carbohydrates with the correct amount of protein (see page 39).

Try this nutritional format for two weeks, then retake your body fat measurement. If you eliminate 1 to 2 pounds of body fat per week, you are doing extremely well and should continue. If you haven't experienced this success, if this is not a comfortable way of eating, or if your results begin to taper off, it is time to try something new. Monitor your food intake with the caloric guidelines on page 192.

Hollywood Heart for the Endomorph

The goal is to continue shrinking fat cells. You have set the stage for some serious results, and over these next four weeks you will build on the foundation you created. With a winning nutritional strategy firmly in place, the second and equally important part of shedding body fat is rooted in your cardiovascular program. During your initiation, you were engaging in cardiovascular exercise six times per week. Continue this frequency. You are going to increase the intensity by elevating your heart rate level. If you are presently exercising at 65 percent of your maximum heart rate, I want you to exercise at 70 percent of your maximum during the first week postinitiation. The second week, strive to maintain your heart rate between 70 percent and 75 percent. In week three postinitiation, maintain the same levels, but insert three 2-minute bursts where you elevate your heart rate to 85 percent of your maximum. In week four, try the interval program described on page 200.

Hollywood Sculpt for the Endomorph

In general, the strategies for the endomorphic male and female are remarkably similar. As you continue to eliminate body fat, you will begin to strategically build up specific areas of your body. Women will create upper body shape to become more of an hourglass, and men will build mass in the shoulders to become more rectangular. While these routines are intended to firm up every muscle group, they are specifically designed to build up your upper body, especially your back and shoulders. You will be toning and contouring your body three days each week using relatively light weights with many repetitions. Both men and women will utilize supersets and giant sets to target the shoulders and back.

Supersets

When a superset is prescribed, it indicates you are targeting a particular muscle group for growth and shape. If a superset is indicated, you will perform one set of exercise A, then a set of exercise B, before stretching the muscle out. By using alternating sets of two exercises, you will stimulate growth and definition.

Giant Sets

A giant set combines three or more exercises. You will perform one set of exercise A, immediately followed by exercise B, then a set of exercise C (then a set of exercises D and E), before stretching the muscle out. By using combinations of exercises to target certain muscles, you will stimulate the greatest possible results in the quickest possible time.

SHAPING AND SCULPTING WORKOUTS FOR THE FEMALE ENDOMORPH

Perform two sets of twenty repetitions. Stretch after each set, superset, or giant set.

WEEK ONE

DAY 1	Page	DAY 2	Page	DAY 3	Page
SUPERSET Lying Side Raise	151	Butt Lift	103	SUPERSET Rear Delt	114
SUPERSET Inner Thigh	96	Arrow	95	SUPERSET Pull-In	109
SUPERSET Incline Fly	120	SUPERSET Bent-Over Row	105	SUPERSET Kickback	130
SUPERSET Tricep Extension	128	SUPERSET Karate Curl	139	SUPERSET Hammer Curl	136
SUPERSET One-Arm Row	106	C Sweep	123	SUPERSET Ball Squat	98
SUPERSET Wings	116	Dip	133	SUPERSET Leg Curl	97
Squeeze	144	Ball Crunch	141	Crunch	145
Penguin	147	Penguin	147	Side Raise	150
Leg Curl	97	Ball Small Sit-Up	142	Leg Curl	97

WEEK TWO

DAY 4	Page	DAY 5	Page	DAY 6	Page
SUPERSET Reverse Lunge	94	GIANT SET Beginner Push-Up	124	SUPERSET Inner Thigh	96
SUPERSET Side Kick	102	GIANT SET Wave	117	SUPERSET Leg Curl	97
SUPERSET Frankenstein	122	GIANT SET Kickout	129	Butt Lift	103
SUPERSET W Shoulders	112	SUPERSET Ball Curl	138	GIANT SET Twisting W	113
SUPERSET Pull-Over	107	SUPERSET Hyperextension	108	GIANT SET Dip	133
SUPERSET Overhead Tri	132	Ball Lunge	101	GIANT SET Cross-Curl	137
Leg Lift	148	Squeeze	144	Ball Crunch	141
Corkscrew	149	Side Raise	150	Penguin	147
Lying Side Raise	151	Ball Small Sit-Up	142	Crossover Crunch	146
Crunch	145				

WEEK THREE

DAY 7	Page	DAY 8	Page	DAY 9	Page
SUPERSET Arrow	95	SUPERSET Cheer	115	SUPERSET Reverse Lunge	94
SUPERSET Calf Raise	99	SUPERSET Tricep Extension	120	SUPERSET Side Kick	102
SUPERSET Squat Curl	134	SUPERSET Decline Push-Up	121	SUPERSET Wings	116
SUPERSET Fly	119	SUPERSET One-Arm Row	106	SUPERSET Kickback	130
SUPERSET Shrug	110	SUPERSET Karate Curl	139	SUPERSET Bent-Over Row	105
SUPERSET Ball Press	131	SUPERSET Lunge	93	SUPERSET Hammer Curl	136
Ball Pike	143	Corkscrew	149	Ball Pike	143
Ball Crunch	141	Leg Lift	148	Side Raise	150
Lying Side Raise	151	Crunch	145	Squeeze	144

	DAY 10	Page		DAY 11	Page		DAY 12	Page
SUPERSET	Ball Push-Up	126	SUPERSET	Rear Delt	114	SUPERSET	Frankenstein	122
	Pull-In	109		Ball Press	131		Kickout	129
SUPERSET	Dip	133	SUPERSET	Incline Fly	120	GIANT SET	One-Arm Row	106
	Squat Curl	134		Pull-Over	107		Wave	117
SUPERSET	Inner Thigh	96	SUPERSET	Butt Lift	103		Squat Curl	134
	Arrow	95		Leg Curl	97		Side Kick	102
	Leg Lift	148		Ball Crunch	141		Ball Pike	143
	Penguin	147		Corkscrew	129		Side Raise	150
	Lying Side Raise	151		Ball Small Sit-Up	142		Squeeze	144

SHAPING AND SCULPTING WORKOUTS FOR THE MALE ENDOMORPH

Perform two sets of twenty repetitions. Stretch after each set, superset or giant set.

WEEK ONE

	DAY 1	Page		DAY 2	Page		DAY 3	Page
SUPERSET	Ball Squat	98	SUPERSET	Reverse Lunge	94	SUPERSET	Decline Push-Up	121
	Lunge	93		Calf Raise	99		Tricep Extension	120
GIANT SET	Fly	119	SUPERSET	Bent-Over Row	105	SUPERSET	Pull-In	109
	W Shoulders	112		Hammer Curl	136		Ball Curl	138
	Dip	133	SUPERSET	Rear Delt	114	SUPERSET	Ball Lunge	101
	One-Arm Row	106		Ball Press	134		Arrow	95
	Corkscrew	149		Ball Crunch	141		Ball Pike	143
	Crossover Crunch	146		Penguin	147		Side Raise	150
	Ball Small Sit-Up	142		Crunch	145		Squeeze	144

WEEK TWO

	DAY 4	Page		DAY 5	Page		DAY 6	Page
	Leg Curl	97	SUPERSET	Ball Squat	98	SUPERSET	One-Arm Row	106
SUPERSET	C Sweep	123		Arrow	95		Squat Curl	134
	Kickback	130	SUPERSET	Incline Fly	120	SUPERSET	Lunge	93
GIANT SET	W Shoulders	112		Kickout	129		Cheer	115
	Shrug	110	SUPERSET	Wings	116	SUPERSET	Ball Push-Up	126
	Karate Curl	139		Cross-Curl	137		Overhead Tri	132
	Leg Lift	148		Ball Pike	143		Ball Crunch	141
	Lying Side Raise	151		Corkscrew	149		Side Raise	150
	Crossover Crunch	146		Crunch	145		Penguin	147

The Final Cut:
The Hollywood Body
Lifestyle

ongratulations! You have put in the effort and the sweat. Six weeks ago, I asked you to make a commitment and a promise to yourself. Now I want you to pause for a brief moment and reflect on that promise and what it has meant to you.

You should feel changes in your energy level, stress level, self-esteem, commitment, focus, drive, and confidence. Analyze your results so far. I am confident that you have made improvements to your overall health. If you continue to eat and exercise as you have in the past six weeks, you will offset or prevent some very serious illnesses, and at the very least ensure that your cardiovascular health is the very best it can be. But I know you are looking for more results, so let's take a look at that.

Your Body Type Final Cut

If you are an ectomorph or an endomorph, chances are that your body has not undergone a complete transformation. Gaining weight is tremendously challenging for the ectomorph; so is losing fat for the endomorph. The postinitiation goal was to create enough shape to move into a comfortable combination of your body type and the mesomorph. This may not have happened yet.

Even if you are a mesomorph and would like to lose a substantial amount of fat, chances are you haven't yet. No matter what your body type, if you would like to lose more body fat, don't continue yet. Instead, repeat the last four weeks. This is not like flunking a grade. You have not failed in any way. Your body simply needs more time to make the kind of dramatic changes you would like to see.

Ectomorphs

If you are an ectomorph trying to add more muscle mass or shape, simply repeat the course of action you used for the last four weeks. Keep your cardiovascular activity limited to the barest minimum for heart health. Consider adding more protein to your nutritional regimen. Perhaps you could eat a protein portion the size of your entire hand at every meal. If you are already doing this, perhaps you could decrease the time between meals and add one more meal consisting of a protein shake. Your strength-training regimen is to repeat the cycle of workout routines and push yourself to use heavier weights. The amount of weight you are able to move will be the best indicator of your progress. Over the next four weeks, you might be able to double the amount of weight you are currently using. After you have finished this next cycle, determine if you have created your desired shape. If not, chances are high that you will have made some amazing progress. You may consider repeating the cycle again. In fact, this program might suit your particular needs better than the six-week program outlined in the remainder of this chapter. You could repeat this cycle indefinitely, experiencing greater results with each passing month.

Endomorphs

If you are an endomorph who would like to lose more body fat, repeat the last four weeks of exercises while striving to reduce the lower half of your body and increase muscular mass and density throughout your upper body to create an hourglass figure (women) or a more rectangular shape (men). Give yourself time. Be very honest about what you have been eating. If you have followed the guidelines and your success rate has been high, that's great. However, your discipline might not be enough to stimulate the rapid changes I would like you to experience over the next four weeks. It may be time to be more exact with how much protein and how many calories your body actually needs to make the changes you desire. If you haven't already done so, you may want to consider using the most stringent nutritional guidelines (see page 192).

Your cardiovascular program can really help you achieve change. Add at least 5 minutes to your cardiovascular sessions every week (if not every session). Work your way up to 1-hour cardiovascular sessions. After one week of 1-hour cardiovascular sessions, add another session. Try doing a 45-minute walk first thing in the morning and another 45-minute walk in the evening. If you are inserting anaerobic bursts, continue to do this on your walks. If you are doing intervals, continue to do so during both of these sessions. Continue your toning and strengthening workouts. This is the only way to create upper body mass to balance your body. Simply repeat the workouts. You may repeat this cycle indefinitely until you come to a point where you feel confident that your shape is either an hourglass or a rectangle. Then continue this chapter.

Mesomorphs

If you are a mesomorph who would like to eliminate more body fat, repeat the four-week program you just finished. Add another day of cardiovascular exercise. Then begin increasing each of these sessions by 5 minutes. After two weeks, you might consider only eating foods from the primary choice lists. Then continue this chapter.

The Hollywood Nutrition Final Cut

Some people do not follow a certain diet or nutritional plan. For them, following the Hollywood nutrition principles would be a breakthrough in itself, and there is no doubt that they will come closer to reaching their goals. But for some people to get results, they must make their nutritional program exact. Most of my celebrity and pro-athlete clients are so focused on and dedicated to their fitness program that they actually need a strict eating regimen. Some other clients are so motivated to attain their goals that they want to do anything and everything they can. Here is all the information you'll need to create a nutritional program that is absolutely perfect for you. Whereas the Hollywood nutrition principles were simple and straightforward, this next step is fairly complex, requiring you to measure your food and count your caloric intake for each meal.

How Much Should You Eat?

For this program, 40 percent of your calories should be derived from protein, 40 percent from carbohydrates, and 20 percent from fat. To determine what and how much you should eat, get out your body fat measurements and your calculator.

You need to determine what your total caloric intake should be per day. The first numbers you want to determine are your weight, your body fat percentage, the number of pounds you have in fat, and the amount of your total weight that is lean muscle mass.

1. To determine the number of pounds you have in fat, multiply your weight by your body fat percentage (place the decimal point in front of this number):

_____ × ._____ = _____
(weight)   (body fat percentage)   (pounds of fat)

2. Subtract your weight from the number of pounds of fat:

_____ – _____ = _____
(weight)   (pounds of fat)   (your lean muscle mass)

Your lean muscle mass is a very important number that includes your bones, organs, hair, and nails. Your lean muscle mass requires protein for fuel. The amount of protein you actually need will depend on your activity level. If you want to lose fat (and are doing weight-bearing exercises three days a week), you need 1 gram of protein per pound of lean muscle mass. If you are performing the body type–specific exercises and are looking to tone or shape your muscles, you need 1.25 grams of protein per pound of lean muscle mass. If you are looking to create size or mass, you need 1.5 grams of protein per pound of lean muscle mass. Determine how many grams of protein you need each day using the following calculations:

- To lose fat: Lean muscle mass _____ × 1.00 = _____ grams of protein per day
- To tone: Lean muscle mass _____ × 1.25 = _____ grams of protein per day
- To gain mass: Lean muscle mass _____ × 1.50 = _____ grams of protein per day

How much protein should you have with each meal?

Would you prefer to eat five times per day or six times per day?

_____

Divide the grams of protein you need _____ ÷ _____ number of meals = _____

The result is the number of grams of protein you should have with each meal.

How many calories should you have each day?

Grams of protein I need per meal _____ × 4 (calories in one gram of protein) = _____

This is the amount of calories you need to derive from protein each time you eat. Multiply this number by 2, because you will want the same number of calories from carbohydrates.

Protein calories _____ × 2 = _____

This is the total number of calories from proteins and carbohydrates, which leaves fat. Carry over the last number, and divide that number by 0.8 (fat calories).

Calories from protein and carbs _____ ÷ 0.8 = _____ (calories per meal)

Multiply by the number of meals _____ (5 or 6) × _____ (calories per meal) = _____.

This is the total number of calories you want to ingest every day.

You now know what and how much you need to be eating, how many times per day you should be eating, and how many calories you should have with each meal. You just saved yourself hundreds of dollars in nutritionist's bills. Counting calories may not be the most exciting task, but it will get you results. Most packaged foods have this information on their labels. When you eat out, however, you will need to be familiar with caloric values so that you can stay within your program. I have provided a list of foods with a corresponding caloric value. Although it is by no means complete, the list does represent the foods that will probably be your primary meal choices. If you find that many of the foods you eat are not on this list, you should either consider changing your eating habits slightly or pick up a book that contains a complete list of foods and their caloric content.

Remember these rules:

1. Never have less than 1,000 calories per day or your body will go into starvation mode.
2. Never have more than 50 grams of protein in one sitting.

Unfortunately, this ruins the equation for some of you. If you have less than 100 pounds of lean muscle mass or more than 200 pounds of lean muscle mass and want to add more, you will need to make some adjustments. If you have less than 100 pounds of lean muscle mass, you will need to eat seven meals per day instead of six. You will need this extra meal to maintain your lean muscle mass and the proper functioning of your vital organs. This should bring you above 1,000 calories and should prevent your body from shifting into starvation mode. If you have more than 200 pounds of lean muscle mass, you need to make a slight adjustment so that you are not consuming over 50 grams of protein per meal. Add an extra meal so that you eat seven meals per day instead of six. Your body needs the protein to be spread out more evenly throughout the day.

Keeping Track of Your Meals

For the first two weeks you are using the caloric method, weigh and measure almost everything you eat. Soon you will know by sight what something weighs, or in the case of liquids, their volume. You will have an idea of your caloric intake when you eat in a restaurant.

Keep a daily journal, noting everything you put in your mouth and what time you ate. This may sound a little obsessive, but you will automatically become more regular and consistent in your eating pattern. You will find it easier to stay within the caloric boundaries of your nutritional program. The table beginning on page 196 provides a list of foods with their corresponding caloric values.

	PORTION	CALORIES
PROTEIN		
Beef	4 oz.	300
Chicken breast	4 oz.	195
Dried beans	$1/4$ cup	160
Eggs	1 large	75
Fish	4 oz.	160
Ham	4 oz.	330
Lamb	4 oz.	300
Lunch meats	2 oz.	160
Nuts and seeds	1 oz.	160
Peanut butter	2 tbsp.	200
Pork	4 oz.	325
Sausage	1 link	120
Shellfish	4 oz.	112
Tofu	3 oz.	60
Turkey	4 oz.	178
Veal	4 oz.	213
CARBOHYDRATES		
Vegetables		
Dark Leafy Green		
Broccoli	$1/2$ cup	10
Collard greens	$1/2$ cup	5
Endive	$1/2$ cup	4
Escarole	$1/2$ cup	4
Kale	$1/2$ cup	15
Mixed greens	$1/2$ cup	30
Mustard greens	$1/2$ cup	7
Romaine lettuce	$1/2$ cup	5
Spinach	$1/2$ cup	5
Turnip greens	$1/2$ cup	5
Watercress	$1/2$ cup	2
Deep Yellow		
Carrots	$1/2$ cup	25
Pumpkin	$1/2$ cup	15
Sweet potato	$1/2$ cup	80
Winter squash	$1/2$ cup	50

	PORTION	CALORIES
Starchy		
Corn	$1/2$ cup	90
Green peas	$1/2$ cup	60
Hominy (grits)	$1/4$ cup	140
Potato	$1/2$ cup	70
Rutabaga	$1/2$ cup	25
Taro	$1/2$ cup	30
Dry Beans and Peas (Legumes)		
Black beans	$1/2$ cup	115
Black-eyed peas	$1/2$ cup	100
Chickpeas	$1/2$ cup	135
Kidney beans	$1/2$ cup	110
Lentils	$1/2$ cup	115
Lima beans	$1/2$ cup	105
Mung beans	$1/2$ cup	105
Navy beans	$1/2$ cup	130
Pinto beans	$1/2$ cup	120
Split peas	$1/2$ cup	115
Other Vegetables		
Artichoke	Whole	60
Asparagus	4 spears	15
Bean and alfalfa sprouts	1 cup	10
Beets	$1/2$ cup	30
Cabbage	$1/2$ cup	10
Cauliflower	$1/2$ cup	10
Celery	$1/2$ cup	10
Cucumber	Whole	35
Eggplant	$1/2$ cup	15
Green beans	$1/2$ cup	20
Green pepper	Whole	20
Lettuce	1 head	20
Mushrooms	$1/2$ cup	10
Okra	$1/2$ cup	20
Onions	$1/2$ cup	30
Radishes	$1/2$ cup	5

	PORTION	CALORIES
Snow peas	½ cup	70
Tomato	½ cup	20
Turnips	½ cup	15
Vegetable juices	8 fl. oz.	60
Zucchini	½ cup	15

Fruits

	PORTION	CALORIES
Apple	1 medium	80
Apricot	3 medium	50
Asian pear	1 medium	100
Blueberries	½ cup	40
Cantaloupe	½ melon	95
Citrus juices	8 fl. oz.	140
Cherries	10 medium	50
Cranberries	½ cup	30
Dates	10 whole	230
Figs	1 large	50
Grapefruit	½ medium	45
Grapes	10 medium	15
Guava	1 medium	45
Honeydew	½ cup	30
Kiwi	1 medium	45
Lemon	1 medium	25
Mango	½ cup	55
Nectarine	1 medium	70
Orange	1 medium	70
Papaya	½ cup	35
Passion fruit	1 medium	25
Peach	1 medium	40
Pear	1 medium	100
Pineapple	½ cup	40
Plantain	3 oz.	100
Plum	1 medium	40
Prunes	10 whole	200
Raisins	½ cup	110
Raspberries	½ cup	30
Rhubarb	½ cup	10

	PORTION	CALORIES
Strawberries	½ cup	25
Tangerine	1 medium	40
Watermelon	½ cup	25

GRAINS

Whole Grain

	PORTION	CALORIES
Brown rice	¼ cup	150
Buckwheat	¼ cup	145
Bulgur	¼ cup	150
Corn tortillas	3 whole	140
Graham crackers	8 pieces	130
Granola	½ cup	190
Oatmeal	1 cup	110
Popcorn	2 tbsp. (unpopped)	150
Pumpernickel bread	1 slice	80
Ready-to-eat cereals	¾ cup	130
Rye bread	1 slice	80
Whole wheat bread	1 slice	70
Whole wheat cereals	1 cup	180
Whole wheat pasta	1 cup (cooked)	175

Enriched Grain

	PORTION	CALORIES
Bagels	½ bagel	100
Cornmeal	¼ cup	130
Crackers	5 pieces	70
English muffin	1 piece	140
Farina	1 cup	115
Flour tortillas	1 piece	130
French bread	1 slice	140
Hamburger and hot dog buns	1 roll	135
Italian bread	2 slices	120
Macaroni	1 cup (cooked)	200
Noodles	1 cup	215

(*continued*)

	PORTION	CALORIES

Enriched Grain (continued)

Pancakes and waffles	2 pieces	200
Pretzels	1 oz.	110
Spaghetti	1 cup (cooked)	200
White bread	1 slice	80
White rice	1/4 cup	150

Grain Products with More Fat or Sugar

Biscuits	1 piece	140
Cake (unfrosted)	1/8 cake	200
Cookie	1 cookie	80
Cornbread	1/5 pan	160
Croissant	1 piece	140
Danish	1 piece	130
Doughnuts (plain)	1 piece	170
Muffin	1 piece	160
Tortilla chips	1 oz.	150

FAT

Fats and Oils

Bacon, salt pork	2 slices	60
Butter	1 tbsp.	100
Cream cheese	2 tbsp.	100
Margarine	1 tbsp.	100
Mayonnaise	1 tbsp.	100
Olive oil	1 tbsp.	120
Salad dressing	2 tbsp.	130
Sour cream	2 tbsp.	60
Vegetable oil	1 tbsp.	120

Dairy

Lowfat milk (1%)	8 fl. oz.	105
Lowfat milk (2%)	8 fl. oz.	120
Skim milk	8 fl. oz.	85
Whole milk	8 fl. oz.	150

	PORTION	CALORIES
Half and half	1 tbsp.	20
Nondairy creamer	1 tbsp.	20
Nondairy creamer with flavor	1 tbsp.	40
Buttermilk	1 tbsp.	25
Lowfat cottage cheese	1/2 cup	120
Cheddar cheese	1 oz.	110
Swiss cheese	1 oz.	90
Cheese spreads	2 tbsp.	100
Lowfat plain yogurt	8 oz.	150
Fat-free yogurt	8 oz.	110
Nonfat frozen yogurt	1/2 cup	100
Fruited yogurt	6 oz.	180
Ice cream	1/2 cup	150
Puddings made with milk	4 oz.	160

Sweets

Frozen fruit bar	1 bar	50
Fruit drinks	8 fl. oz.	125
Gelatin desserts	1/2 cup	80
Hard candy	3 pieces	70
Honey	1 tbsp.	60
Jam	1 tbsp.	50
Jelly	1 tbsp.	50
Maple syrup	1/4 cup	210
Marmalade	1 tbsp.	60
Molasses	1 tbsp.	60
Sherbet	1/2 cup	120
Soft drinks and colas	8 fl. oz.	100
Sugar (brown)	1 oz.	110
Sugar (white)	1 tbsp.	50

Alcoholic Beverages

Beer	12 fl. oz.	150
Liquor	1 fl. oz.	65
Wine	1 fl. oz.	25

The Hollywood Heart Final Cut

You can do only so much to eliminate fat with nutrition alone. Most of your fat-loss results will be derived from cardiovascular activity. To really push this, add one extra day of cardiovascular activity per week (unless you are an ectomorph). Always remember to take one day off each week to allow your body to rest and rejuvenate. In addition, increase the duration and intensity of your cardiovascular sessions. Add at least 5 minutes to each of your sessions. Then increase the duration of each session by an additional 5 minutes each week. When these sessions build up to 1 hour, simply continue if you are happy with the results. If you want to lose even more body fat or have another fitness goal, you may exercise up to six days per week, and you may also do two cardiovascular sessions each day. If you add a second session each day, limit each session to 45 minutes.

The Hollywood Sculpt Final Cut

As more and more body fat is eliminated, the muscles underneath will begin to appear. The next six weeks of your program will shape and contour each muscle.

Hollywood Heart

Here is a finishing program to bring your heart health up to optimal levels and to dramatically reduce body fat. This program begins with walking. (Don't forget to buy a heart rate monitor. It is money well spent.) Always keep in mind that you must surprise your body to get results. If you perform the exact same routine day after day, your body will quickly adapt and expend the least amount of energy possible. If you are walking outdoors, take a different route every day or every other day. If you can, choose a route that has varying terrain (hills, inclines, or steps).

For the first two weeks, increase your heart rate to 70 percent and walk for at least 25 minutes every day. The more you use your arms when you walk, the greater your heart rate. This daily walk will become a ritual. It will be the portion of your day when you allow yourself to think. You can also share this time—bring along a friend or family member, your dog, or a colleague from the office. You will be surprised by the quality and productivity of this time.

In week three, continue to walk for at least 25 consecutive minutes, but walk only six days this week. Choose three days to do a little more cardiovascular work so that you elevate your heart rate to 80 to 85 percent for five 1-minute spurts. After the minute is over, decrease your arm movement and/or slow your pace to reduce your heart rate level to 70 percent. These bursts should quickly increase your fitness level so that you are ready for some serious fat-burning cardiovascular sessions.

In week four, you are going to change your routine ever so slightly. At the end of this week, you will have formed a positive addiction, a new behavioral habit of regular exercise. Chances are that you have experienced an increase in energy level, a reduction of stress, clear-headedness, and a renewed sense of vitality. During this week, your cardiovascular session will solidify into a habit that you simply cannot do without.

Get your heart rate up to 85 percent and keep it there for 2 minutes, and perform five of these 2-minute bursts every time you do your cardiovascular exercise. It may take some effort to get your heart rate to reach 85 percent of your maximum. You may really have to pick up the pace, maximize the involvement of your arms, bring along a set of light dumbbells, or jog. In addition to burning more body fat, you will increase your fitness level and strengthen your heart muscle. During the entire week, extend your workout session an additional 5 minutes so that you are performing at least 30 minutes of cardiovascular exercise every day. By the end of this fourth week, you will be ready for new challenges.

In week five, you will do interval training, varying your heart rate every 2 minutes. Begin your session by walking at a comfortable pace, elevating your heart rate to 60 percent of your maximum for 2 minutes. Then increase your heart rate to 70 percent for 2 minutes. For the next 2 minutes, elevate your heart rate to 80 percent of your maximum. Return to the 70 percent level for the next 2 minutes, and alternate between the 70 and 80 percent levels in these 2-minute blocks for at least 30 minutes. During this week, you may choose to increase the duration of your cardiovascular exercise by another 5 minutes. Even if you feel like you could increase the duration of your session by 10 minutes, don't overdo it this week. You can experience burnout, and your body and mind can begin to resist regular cardiovascular exercise if you push too hard.

During week six, something miraculous might happen. The more active you are, the more active you will become, and during this week you just might discover yourself finding time for even more activity. This could start small—for example, playing a set or two of tennis, going for a nature hike, playing ball with the neighborhood kids, or trying some kind of activity that you have always wanted to try. There will be a noticeable increase in your desire to become more active, and when you get the desire, go for it. To support this momentum, increase the duration of your intervals, and increase the duration of your cardiovascular sessions. Alternate between 70 and 80 percent of your maximum heart rate in 3-minute intervals, and increase your sessions by another 5 minutes so that you are performing at least 40 minutes of cardiovascular activity. After you complete this week of cardiovascular training, it is time to reevaluate your goals.

Continue if you feel this level of activity suits your needs and fits within your schedule. Remember to choose a different route every other day so that you are not on the same terrain for two consecutive days. Stay with the 3-minute intervals, and alternate between 70 and 80 percent of your maximum heart rate.

If you want to shake things up or if you want to increase your heart health and fitness level even further, occasionally (no more than twice per session) get your heart rate near the 90 percent range for 10 seconds. You may also increase the duration of each session, but try to increase it by only 5 minutes, and wait a full week before bumping it up another 5 minutes. Push yourself to extend the jogging portion of your interval. In no time at all, you will be jogging the entire session, and you will have to pick up your pace to reach that 80 percent rate. You may even set your sights on training for a 5k or 10k race. Unless you are training for such an event, you will have maximized the session after about an hour. After $1^{1}/_{2}$ hours, you will get no further benefits. If you ever happen to get to the place where you can do your interval training for $1^{1}/_{2}$ hours, you have indeed become a healthy addict, and you may consider doing one hour in the morning and another hour in the evening.

Other Cardiovascular Activities

If you feel that interval walking is not for you, you may want to look at doing something that might be more exciting. There are many activities that will do as much if not more for your heart health and enable you to burn even more body fat. Sometimes it takes a little experimentation to discover what activity suits you best. If you would prefer to exercise indoors, you can go into virtually any gym or sports club facility to discover many fun and exciting options for cardiovascular activity. If you like to exercise outdoors, the options are almost limitless.

If you choose an outdoor activity, the only rule is to do 40 consecutive minutes of exercise six days per week. Continue to interval train, alternating between 70 and 80 percent of your maximum heart rate in 3-minute intervals. You may want to jump rope outdoors and take in the sun, or ride your bike, varying terrain so that your body does not become used to the workout. You may live near a river where people row in skulls (an amazingly fun and challenging workout). Swimming is a very beneficial choice because you truly work every muscle group to elevate your heart rate, and you use resistance and stretching techniques with every stroke. Swimming does not put stress on the joints, limiting the possibility of injury.

At the gym you will find many options to complete your cardio-vascular exercise. Many gyms offer aerobics classes. These are not what they used to be; they have gone through a significant evolution and have adapted many disciplines. There are classes that stress high impact, low impact, jazzercise, hip-hop, country western, resistance aerobics, kickboxing, aerobics using an elevated step, spinning (aerobics performed on a stationary bike), and even water aerobics. In addition to being a lot of fun, these classes are supervised and are offered frequently to fit into your schedule. Most gyms are equipped with stationary bikes, rowing machines, step machines, ski machines, treadmills, climbers, and elliptical trainers.

The Rowing Machine

The rowing machine is a fantastic device to achieve a cardiovascular workout. It requires you to use many if not all of your body's muscle groups. Although rowing is one of the most effective forms of cardiovascular exercise, it is the least likely to sustain your interest for long.

For the best results on this machine, you should vary the intensity of your rowing pace. You may begin at a relatively relaxed pace to bring your heart rate up to the 60 percent range, and after a few minutes take it up to 70 percent. At the 10-minute mark, begin to perform your interval training. Do this by increasing your heart rate to 80 or 85 percent for 2 minutes, and bring it back down to 70 percent for 3 minutes. Five minutes before the end of your exercise session, reduce your heart rate to 60 percent. Each day you exercise on the rowing machine, begin the interval training 30 seconds sooner. After only a short time, you will be starting your interval training at the 1-minute mark. When you have reached this point, begin extending the intervals at which you achieve 85 percent of your maximum heart rate by 15 seconds, and decrease by 15 seconds the portion of the interval where you are at 70 percent of your maximum heart rate.

The Stationary Bike

The stationary bike is one of the most used machines at the gym, and in my opinion, one of the least effective at giving you a sufficient cardiovascular workout, primarily because the entire upper portion of your body is not in motion. When you are walking or jogging, rowing or skiing, the arms are swinging or moving. As a result, the heart must be called upon to pump blood to these limbs, increasing both your circulation and heart rate.

If you use the stationary bike, you should always create arm movement. Pump your arms, use 1- or 2-pound dumbbells for curls and an assortment of tricep exercises, or even try boxinglike motions with your arms to involve your upper body and increase your heart rate. If you do not involve your arms with some kind of motion, you will have to pedal furiously to get your heart rate up, and you may not finish your cardiovascular workout. If you do involve the arms, it is best to select a random course setting that will effectively raise and lower the intensity of resistance. The random course will simulate riding up and down an assortment of hills and ask you to increase and decrease your speed. Most computerized stationary bikes have a number of course selections, and you should use a different course each time you exercise on this machine. If the stationary bike you are using does not have computerized controls, simply increase and decrease the resistance level in specific time intervals, changing those intervals each time you exercise on that machine.

The Treadmill

The treadmill is an excellent machine to take you into your aerobic target zone. This machine is best utilized by not holding onto the handrails. Like the stationary bike, the treadmill is maximized when you can involve the upper half of your body. When you walk or jog on the treadmill and do not hold onto the handrails, your arms will naturally swing back and forth. Like many other cardio-vascular machines at the gym, a computer often controls the tread-mill. The computer controls will increase the incline level you are walking or jogging on to simulate the experience of going up and down hills. There are a number of courses to choose from, with a wide array of speeds. Make a note of what you did today and do a different course tomorrow.

The Step Machine

The step machine, commonly known as the StairMaster, is a fine choice to give you an excellent cardiovascular workout. While some find this a difficult workout, it is actually my personal preference. Like the stationary bike and the treadmill, this machine is most effective when you can involve your arms. Many people who have used this machine complain that it is not effective. Many people also use it incorrectly because they hold onto the handrails and let their arms support most of their weight. Used correctly, these handrails should only give you balance. If you can avoid using the handrails altogether, this machine actually provides a challenging and invigorating cardiovascular workout.

Whereas exercising on the treadmill provides periods when you are walking or jogging over a flat terrain, the step machine always simulates the experience of going uphill. Choose a different com-puterized course each day to get the greatest results. Aside from pro-viding a great sweat, this machine can bring definition to the calves, the thighs, and the gluteal (butt) muscles.

The Elliptical Trainer

The elliptical trainer is arguably the finest possible choice of gym equipment to meet your needs. It combines the best attributes of all the machines into one effective device. The footrests are designed to move in the shape of a football—that is, in a sort of oval shape. Because of this design, the machine is low impact, reducing the risk of injury to the knees and joints.

The elliptical trainer is usually equipped with the most sophisticated computer, that regulates the incline level in an almost endless array of courses. Each course selection can be quite different and ensures that you will not become bored. The elliptical trainer gives you the low-impact workout you would get on the stationary bike, simulates the walking or jogging motion that you would enjoy on the treadmill, and trains over a hilly terrain not unlike the step machine.

In addition to providing a fantastic workout that eliminates the possibility of injury, the elliptical trainer develops and defines the musculature in the thighs, calves, and buttocks. You must consciously involve the arms when using this machine. The more movement in your arms, the greater the circulation. And, of course, the greater the circulation, the greater the health benefits associated with cardiovascular exercise.

As this program kicks into a higher gear, you will see changes unfold at a rapid pace. You will continue to lose body fat and should see the muscles more clearly. You may exceed every expectation that you had for yourself. If you have not yet reached your goal, it is well within your attainment.

HOLLYWOOD FINAL CUT FOR WOMEN

Perform two sets of fifteen repetitions. Stretch after each set or superset.

WEEK ONE

DAY 1	Page	DAY 2	Page	DAY 3	Page
Incline Fly	120	Arrow	95	Frankenstein	122
Rear Delt	114	Inner Thigh	96	Pull-In	109
Kickback	130	Butt Lift	103	Wings	116
Bent-Over Row	105	Wave	117	Reverse Lunge	94
Squat Curl	134	Tricep Extension	128	Leg Curl	97
Crossover Crunch	146	Ball Crunch	141	Leg Lift	148
Side Raise	150	Lying Side Raise	151	Corkscrew	149
Ball Small Sit-Up	142	Squeeze	144	Crunch	145

WEEK TWO

DAY 4	Page	DAY 5	Page	DAY 6	Page
Lunge	93	Fly	119	Cheer	115
Arrow	95	Dip	133	Tricep Extension	128
Side Kick	102	Twisting W	113	Pull-Over	107
SUPERSET Beginner Push-Up	124	One-Arm Row	106	Butt Lift	103
SUPERSET Rear Delt	114	Ball Squat	98	SUPERSET Ball Lunge	101
Overhead Tri	132	Arrow	95	SUPERSET Calf Raise	99
Ball Pike	143	Corkscrew	149	Ball Pike	143
Penguin	147	Leg Lift	148	Side Raise	150
Crunch	145	Squeeze	144	Ball Small Sit-Up	142

WEEK THREE

DAY 7	Page	DAY 8	Page	DAY 9	Page
C Sweep	123	Lunge	93	Incline Fly	120
Shrug	110	Arrow	95	Dip	133
Wave	117	Calf Raise	99	Twisting W	113
Side Kick	102	SUPERSET Wings	116	Squat Curl	134
Inner Thigh	96	SUPERSET Ball Press	131	Inner Thigh	96
Leg Curl	97	Leg Lift	148	Reverse Lunge	94
Ball Crunch	141	Lying Side Raise	151	Corkscrew	149
Corkscrew	149	Crossover Crunch	146	Side Raise	150
Crunch	145			Ball Crunch	141

WEEK FOUR

DAY 10	Page	DAY 11	Page	DAY 12	Page
SUPERSET Ball Squat	98	Frankenstein	122	Butt Lift	103
SUPERSET Side Kick	102	Hyperextension	108	Lunge	93
Butt Lift	103	Bent-Over Row	105	SUPERSET Incline Fly	120
Rear Delt	114	Wave	117	SUPERSET Wings	116
Kickback	130	Arrow	95	One-Arm Row	106
Cross-Curl	137	Leg Curl	97	Overhead Tri	132
Ball Pike	143	Crossover Crunch	146	Ball Curl	138
Lying Side Raise	151	Corkscrew	149	Ball Crunch	141
Leg Lift	148	Crunch	145	Penguin	147
				Squeeze	144

Perform two sets of fifteen repetitions. Stretch after each set or superset.

WEEK ONE

DAY 1	Page	DAY 2	Page	DAY 3	Page
Advanced Push-Up	125	Lunge	93	Leg Curl	97
Bent-Over Row	105	Arrow	95	Squat Curl	134
Rear Delt	114	Decline Push-Up	121	Overhead Tri	132
Ball Press	131	W Shoulders	112	One-Arm Row	106
Ball Curl	138	Dip	133	Ball Push-Up	126
Ball Squat	98	Karate Curl	139	Wings	116
Leg Lift	148	Ball Pike	143	Ball Crunch	141
Corkscrew	149	Side Raise	150	Squeeze	144
Crunch	145	Corkscrew	149	Crossover Crunch	146

WEEK TWO

DAY 4	Page	DAY 5	Page	DAY 6	Page
Dip	133	Lunge	93	Ball Push-Up	126
Frankenstein	122	Arrow	95	Pull-Over	107
Pull-In	109	C Sweep	123	Shrug	110
Wave	117	Twisting W	113	Rear Delt	114
Hammer Curl	136	Ball Press	131	Kickback	130
Lunge	93	Ball Curl	138	Karate Curl	139
Leg Lift	148	Ball Pike	143	Ball Squat	98
Lying Side Raise	151	Leg Lift	148	Corkscrew	149
Penguin	147	Crossover Crunch	146	Side Raise	150
				Ball Crunch	141

WEEK THREE

DAY 7	Page	DAY 8	Page	DAY 9	Page
Reverse Lunge	94	Fly	119	Twisting W	113
Leg Curl	97	Kickout	129	Dip	133
W Shoulders	112	Wave	117	Pull-Over	107
Bent-Over Row	105	Squat Curl	134	Karate Curl	139
Tricep Extension	128	Lunge	93	Reverse Lunge	94
Hammer Curl	136	Calf Raise	99	Leg Curl	97
Crunch	145	Ball Crunch	141	Leg Lift	148
Lying Side Raise	151	Corkscrew	149	Ball Pike	143
Squeeze	144	Penguin	147	Ball Small Sit-Up	142

SUPERSET	DAY 10	Page	DAY 11	Page	SUPERSET	DAY 12	Page
⎰	Arrow	95	Lunge	93	**⎰**	Fly	119
⎱	Squat Curl	134	Leg Curl	97	**⎱**	Wave	117
	Decline Push-Up	121	One-Arm Row	106		Tricep Extension	128
	Rear Delt	114	C Sweep	123		Ball Curl	138
	Overhead Tri	132	Cheer	115		Reverse Lunge	94
	Hyperextension	108	Kickback	130		Calf Raise	99
	Ball Crunch	141	Ball Pike	143		Leg Lift	148
	Side Raise	150	Corkscrew	149		Crossover Crunch	146
	Squeeze	144	Crossover Crunch	146		Squeeze	144

What Next?

would like you now to acknowledge exactly how much you have done for yourself and how far you have come. I want you to know just how powerful you are. I want you to feel proud, and completely empowered by what you have done.

Take a deep breath. Relax. Pat yourself on the back. Feel the satisfaction that comes from a job well done. Take a look around you. Look at your living environment, your job, and your important relationships. Do you see the improvements? Take a look at your physical appearance. Are there any improvements in the way you dress, your grooming, or the pride you take in your presentation? Take a look at your life and give credit where credit is due. It wasn't me. I didn't wave a magic wand over your life. I merely gave you a road map to make things different. You did all the work. You put in the effort, carved out the time, and had the focus and discipline.

In changing your body, you may have changed your life. Like throwing a pebble into a still pond, the changes you have made and your new mindset will have a ripple effect throughout the rest of your life. Each of those ripples will become a wave. The more time passes and the longer you continue on this path, the greater the momentum, and each of those waves will become larger. You have done something very significant. You have embarked on a path that has changed and will continue to change your life. As you continue on that path, you should now determine your next step.

Truly you have only just begun. My goal is still for you to maintain a healthy and active lifestyle. Exercising and healthy eating are becoming second nature to you. I hope you feel so good that you will never consider reverting to your previous lifestyle patterns. These healthy new habits have positively addicted you to a great way of living.

What would you like to do next? The choices are limitless. You could repeat the cycle of workouts over and over again. If you would like to improve further, you could take another step. By this time, you are fit enough to do just about anything you choose. You could take up a new sport or activity. Perhaps you would like to weight train more extensively to create even more shape, strength, tone, and muscle mass or density. If so, I have a terrific audio program that is exactly like having me as your personal trainer at the gym. If you need some ideas, check out my Web site at www.atighteru.com. You will see new workout routines and additional exercises, find ideas to increase fitness and build upon your results, locate trainers or facilities in your area, or have your questions answered by e-mail.

If you have experienced results and are satisfied with the progress you have made thus far, my suggestion is to simply continue what you are doing. If you continue, you are in the top 10 percent of the most active and fit people in North America!

Above all, my philosophy is to keep it simple. Your nutrition program should be as easy as you can make it. Using hand measurements to determine protein portion sizes along with the proper ratio of carbohydrates will now suit your needs. Continue your cardiovascular program and continue to do what you are already doing. If you want to challenge yourself or push yourself toward greater results you can increase the intensity and duration of your cardiovascular session. At most, you can do two cardiovascular sessions per day, and these sessions can last up to one hour. You can do this up to six days per week. The six-week toning program you just completed can be used again and again. If you would like to increase the number of days you work out, by all means do so. You can strength train up to six days per week, in which case this is a three-week program, not a six-week program.

I preach the virtues of exercise and proper eating all day, every day. And I practice what I preach. I watch what I eat and exercise a great deal because I truly believe that it is the key to living a full life. The more disciplined I become, the more value I see in the investment of time and effort. It is what gives my life the greatest meaning and the greatest purpose. My hope is that it will become this meaningful to you.

It is now time to reward yourself. Maybe you would like to take a vacation and show off your Hollywood body on some exotic beach. If this fits the bill, just make sure you purchase something on your trip to remind you of that place and the purpose of the trip. In the military, people are given medals for achievement. Some people get a tattoo to mark a rite of passage. When you graduate from college, you receive a diploma. You need to give yourself something equally significant to remind you of your accomplishment.

After doing what you have just done, many people find that their clothes no longer fit. As a reward and out of necessity, they treat themselves to new clothing. This is an excellent commemoration of your hard work and effort. If you choose this as your reward or if you are forced to choose this reward because your clothes don't fit, start with only the essentials. Give yourself further motivation to stick with this program by setting up a reward system. Just as people who are in Alcoholics Anonymous are awarded a medallion to indicate how many days, months, or years they have been sober, you should get a new article of clothing to add to your wardrobe every week.

Set up small goals for yourself. You want to continue eating healthy. You want to continue your cardiovascular exercise. You want to continue to tone, shape, and sculpt. After every completed week, get yourself a little something to add to your new wardrobe—a shirt, a pair of pants, a skirt. For every completed month, make it more extensive. Perhaps it could be a stunning new outfit for the office or evenings out; perhaps an assortment of casual clothes. Celebrate in a big way every three months, and again make this shopping excursion something special—perhaps a new and essential seasonal clothing package, a new set of clothes for work, or a special suit or dress. After two (three-month) seasons, chances are very high that you will never again wear the clothes you wore when you started this program. After your second seasonal shopping spree, take time to collect all of the clothes that are now too big and find a place that can use them. To celebrate your new body and your new life, give your old clothes away to a worthy person, group, or institution. In doing so, you have said good-bye to your former physique and given your new self a grand new entrance.

Index

Flockhart, Calista, 12, 156
Fly, 119
Frankenstein, 122
free foods, 38–39, 79
  selections for, 38
front stretch, 93, 94, 101
fruit, 79

Garner, Jennifer, 157
giant sets, 172
  for endomorphs, 182
glucose, 35
  body's use of, 51
  lowering, in bloodstream, 75
Goodman, John, 157
green tea, 78, 80

habits
  acquisition of healthy new, 214
  establishing new, 73
  solidifying good, 200
Hammer Curl, 136
heart principles, 25, 45–56
  aerobic and anaerobic exercise, 47–48
  exercise, 46–47, 51–56. *See also* cardiovas-
    cular exercise; exercise
  getting aerobic, 49
  monitoring heart rate, 50–51
  walking, 54–56
heart rate
  aerobic level for, 49
  calculating ideal, 49
  elevating, 47, 49, 54, 200
  monitoring, 50–51
  near 90 percent range, 202
  varying, 201
  walking, and raising of, 55–56

heart rate monitors, 50–51, 83–84,
    199
Hilton, Paris, 156, 179
hips, 100
  Ball Lunge, 101
  Butt Lift, 103
  exercises, 101–103
  Side Kick, 102
hip stretch, 102, 103
Hollywood body system
  background, 1–5
  initiation, 73–91
  Web site, 158, 214
Hurley, Elizabeth, 157
hydrostatic weighing, 30
Hyperextension, 108

imbalance, 21
  determining muscular, 23
immune system, boosting, 61
Incline Fly, 120
infrared imaging, 3, 62–63, 65
initiation
  completing, 152
  first two weeks, 73–91
  heart, 81–86
  for men, toning, 91
  nutrition, 74–76
  sculpt, 86–90
  structure of programs in, 155
  for women, toning, 90–91
Inner Thigh, 96
insulin, 35
  secretion of, 75

Jackson, Janet, 140
Jagger, Mick, 156

jogging
  and burning of calories, 55
  heart rate and, 202
  on treadmill, 204–205
  varying pace of, 52–53
  varying terrain for, 53
journal, keeping, 40, 195
jumping rope, 202
junk food, 77

Karate Curl, 139
ketosis, 75
  leading body into state of, 80
  products that take you out of, 81
Kickback, 130
Kickout, 129

lactic acid
  buildup, 53
  flushing out, 67, 90
Lao-tzu, 11
latissimus dorsi muscles, 22
lean muscle mass, 86–87, 193
  increasing, 61, 86
  number of meals to eat and, 195
Leg Curl, 97
Leg Lift, 148
legs, 21
  Arrow, 95
  Ball Squat, 98
  Calf Raise, 99
  creating symmetric balance in, 60, 66–67
  exercises for, 93–99
  Inner Thigh, 96
  Leg Curl, 97
  Lunge, 93
  Reverse Lunge, 94
lifestyle
  acknowledging healthy, 213–216

active, 1–2
changes in, 73–74
rewarding yourself for new, 215–216
Lopez, Jennifer, 100, 118, 157, 179
low blood sugar, effects of, 80–81
Lunge, 93
Lying Side Raise, 151

Madonna, 157
Maguire, Tobey, 59, 156
Manheim, Camryn, 12
meals
  amount of protein and vegetables for, 79
  brushing teeth after, 40
  keeping track of, 195
  necessary, to maintain lean muscle mass, 195
  number of, 39
  planning, 40, 74
  and portion size, 35–39
  in restaurants, 39–40, 81
  snack-size, 34
  timing of, 76
men
  achieving finely toned chest for, 118
  arms of, 23–24
  body fat formula for, 31–32
  ectomorph, 156
  endomorph, 157, 181–182, 191
  Final Cut for, 208–209
  mesomorph, 157, 169
  minimal amount of body fat necessary for, 32
  prototypes of bodies desired by, 59
  reshaping body type of, 158
  shapely buttocks for, 100
  shaping and sculpting workouts for ectomorph, 165–166

men (*continued*)

  shaping and sculpting workouts for endomorph, 184–185

  shaping and sculpting workouts for mesomorph, 174–175

  symbolization of arms to, 127

  toning initiation for, 91

mesomorphs, 15, 157

  cardiovascular exercise for, 170–171

  challenges for, 190

  Final Cut program for, 191–192

  giant sets for, 172

  nutrition for, 170

  physical characteristics of, 169

  sculpt principles for, 171–172

  shaping and sculpting workouts for female, 173–174

  shaping and sculpting workouts for male, 174–175

  supersets for, 172

metabolism

  accelerating, 61

  creating new baseline for, 76, 78

  of ectomorphs, 161

  resetting, 14, 41, 73

  speeding up, 46

  supercharging, 47

mitochondria, burning, 47–48

momentumless training, 64–68

  breathing, 65–66

  stretching, 67–68

  using principles of, 89–90

Moss, Kate, 156

multivitamins, 78

muscles

  achieving 100 percent of capability of, 65

  core, 140

  definition, 59

  development of back, 104

  infrared imaging of, 3, 62–63, 65

  mass, gaining, 36, 61

  primary, 63

  secondary, 63

  soreness of, 90

  stretching, 67–68

  tertiary, 63

  tissue, 62

  tone, 59

  utilization of amino acids by lean, 35

  warming up, 47

  weight of, 86

Norton, Edward, 156, 179

nutrition principles, 25, 29–41

  body fat, 29–32

  combining proteins and carbohydrates, 34–39

  for ectomorphs, 162

  for endomorphs, 180–181

  Final Cut, 192–195

  food selection, 77

  helpful tips, 80–81

  initiation phase, 74–76

  limiting or avoiding stimulants, 77–78

  for mesomorphs, 170

  new eating program, 78–80

  outthinking your body, 33–34

  portion size, 35–39

  reminders, hints, and tricks, 39–40

  timing and, 76

One-Arm Row, 106

osteoporosis, combating, 46

Overhead Tri, 132

pectoral muscles, 23, 119

Penguin, 147
physiology, 3
Pitt, Brad, 59, 156
portions, size of, 35–39
posture, 22, 23
    effect of imbalances on, 21
    -related ailments, 87
primary carbohydrates, 36, 38
    selections for, 37
primary muscle, 63
primary proteins, 36
    selections for, 37
proteins
    amino acids derived from, 35
    and carbohydrates, combining, 34–39
    choices of secondary, 36
    choosing, 78–79
    determining grams of, 193–194
    portion size of, 36
    primary, selections for, 37
Pull-In, 109
Pull-Over, 107
pulse
    accurately measuring, 50
    finding, 50

quadricep muscles, 92

ragdoll stretch, 95, 97, 98
random weight, loss of, 33–34
Rear Delt, 114
repetitions, 63
    difficulty of last few, 65
    muscle performance during first several, 64
    number of, and weight training, 68
resistance training, 61
    with active stretching, 67–68

restaurants, meals in, 39–40, 81
    and knowing caloric food values, 194
Reverse Lunge, 94
rowing, 202
rowing machines, 203–204

Schwarzenegger, Arnold, 157
sculpt principles, 25, 59–70
    body symmetry, 60
    for ectomorphs, 162–163
    for endomorphs, 181–182
    exercise vocabulary, 63
    Final Cut, 199
    initiation, 86–90
    logic of sculpting, 62–63
    for mesomorphs, 171–172
    momentumless training, 64–68
    strategy, 59–60
    strength planning, 87
    timing of toning, 87–88
    toning and shaping, 61
    weight training tips, 68–70
secondary carbohydrates, 36
    selections for, 38
secondary muscle, 63
    involvement, eliminating, 64
secondary proteins, 36
self-esteem, increasing, 10, 70
sets, 63. See also giant sets; supersets
    active stretching between, 67–68
    number of, and weight training, 68
shaping, 61
    and sculpting workouts for female ectomorphs, 164–165
    and sculpting workouts for female endomorphs, 183–184
    and sculpting workouts for female mesomorphs, 173–174

toning
   initiation for men, 91
   initiation for women, 90–91
   muscle, 59
   and shaping, 61
   strategies, 68–69
   timing of, 87–88
   Zen of, 88
trapezius muscles, 22
treadmills, 204–205
   varying incline level of, 52, 53
Tricep Extension, 128
tricep muscles, 24
   exercises for, 128–133
   highly developed, 127
tricep stretch, 128, 129, 130, 131, 132, 133
Twisting W, 113
Tyler, Steven, 156

vegetables, 41, 79
vocabulary, exercise, 63

walking, 54–56, 199–201
   guidelines, 84–85
   varying terrain for, 53
water, 90
   benefits of drinking lots of, 80
   loss of, 33–34
   necessary minimum amount of, 40
Wave, 117
weight
   gain, inactivity and, 46
   loss, as goal, 12
weight lifting, 48, 64–68. *See also* weight
   training

weight training
   benefits of, 61
   offsetting aging process with, 61
   and stretching, 67–68
   tips, 68–70
   See also weight lifting
well-being, achieving feelings of, 11
Willis, Bruce, 157
Winfrey, Oprah, 157
Wings, 116
women
   achieving finely toned chest for,
      118
   arms of, 23–24
   body fat formula for, 30–31
   ectomorph, 156
   endomorph, 157, 181–182, 191
   Final Cut for, 206–207
   mesomorph, 157, 169
   minimal amount of body fat necessary for,
      32
   prototypes of bodies desired by, 59
   reshaping body type of, 158
   shapely buttocks for, 100
   shaping and sculpting workouts for ecto-
      morph, 164–165
   shaping and sculpting workouts for endo-
      morph, 183–184
   shaping and sculpting workouts for meso-
      morph, 173–174
   symbolization of arms to, 127
   toning initiation for, 90–91
W Shoulders, 112

Zellweger, Renee, 2
Zen, 88
Zeta-Jones, Catherine, 12